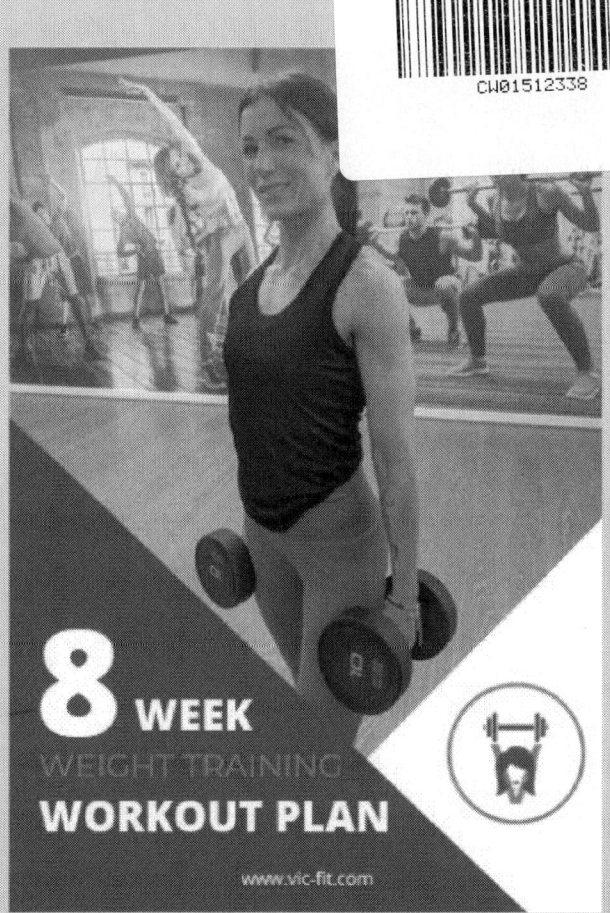

CW01512338

8 WEEK

WEIGHT TRAINING

WORKOUT PLAN

www.vic-fit.com

Would you like my 8-week gym workout plan for free? Grab your copy at: **www.vic-fit.com**

Stronger Than Ever

A Woman's Guide To Physical & Mental Strength Through Weight Training

By Victoria Murphy

Copyright 2020 Victoria Murphy

All rights reserved

Author's Legal Disclaimer

This book is solely for informational and educational purposes and is not medical advice. Please consult a medical or health professional before you begin any new exercise, nutrition or supplementation programme, or if you have questions about your health.

Always put safety first when lifting weights in the gym. Any use of the information within this book is at the reader's discretion and risk.

The author cannot be held responsible for any loss, claim or damage arising out of the use, or misuse, of the suggestions made, the failure to take medical advice, or for any related material from third party sources.

No part of this publication shall be reproduced, transmitted, or sold in any form without the prior written consent of the author.

All trademarks and registered trademarks appearing in this book are the property of their respective owners.

Table of Contents

Introduction

"Weight training?"

"To lose weight?"

"Are you f*cking kidding me?"

Three short sentences I'm guessing ran through your mind the first time you considered lifting weights to get in shape.

How do I know? I had these exact thoughts six years ago. That's when I was:

- Overweight and out of shape
- Jumping from one fad diet to another
- Trying every new exercise trend ever invented
- Obsessed with finding something that actually worked for fat loss
- Feeling I was hitting a brick wall with every attempt to get in shape
- Pretending to feel happy and content with myself

I could go on a while here.

It made no sense at the time that lifting weights could result in fat loss and better tone. Up until that point I was convinced that women and weights = big and bulky.

If you thought that too, then we were both wrong. But I'm guessing you've figured that out by now - and that's why you've picked up this book.

But what exercises should you do? How many times a week should you train? What should you eat? How much weight should you lift? Should you get a personal trainer? Should you count your calories? Do you need to eat loads of protein?

Just some of the many questions I imagine have been on your mind.

Those questions – and so many more - are about to be answered. This book provides a straightforward path to your fitness goals, whether you're a complete beginner or have been a gym member for a while, getting nowhere.

And we all know that diet is the area where most of us struggle, and that's why this book has three chapters dedicated to a simplified way of eating.

So, that doesn't mean counting calories. It doesn't mean heavily restricting your diet. And it certainly doesn't mean struggling to eat healthy all the time.

In fact, if you follow what I'm about to teach in this book, you'll get to the stage where you can freely enjoy your food – and have a better relationship with it.

But why listen to me? I've been where you likely are now. Six years ago I hadn't even considered picking up a dumbbell. Honestly, I was completely terrified about venturing into the weights section in the gym.

I'll explain soon exactly how I made that first crucial step. But safe to say, it's been one of the most important steps of my entire life. I've gone from being overweight, unhealthy and unhappy to confident, content and stronger than I ever imagined.

I've spent the past six years developing my body and mind through my dedication to weight training and adopting a new healthier lifestyle. I've made many mistakes, gained tons of knowledge, and experimented with various training systems along the way.

After more than 1,000 gym workouts, countless sets of exercises, and an intense love for the gym, I now have a refined approach to weight training that's applicable to women of all ages, shapes and sizes – and is guaranteed to get you results in the gym. (As long as you put in the work).

I know this for a fact as many friends have had similar success as me by using this approach.

I'm not a gym instructor. I'm not a personal trainer. I'm not a nutritionist or dietitian. I'm an Advanced Nurse Practitioner and weight training started off as my hobby...but then became an obsession.

In the past six years of lifting weights in the gym, and constantly educating myself on health and diet, I have discovered a fitness lifestyle that works for women. I've written this book to share the best of everything I've learned with you.

We all get started on our fitness journey for results, but the results through weight training and the methods I teach in this book go way beyond what you'd expect.

Yes, you will absolutely lose bodyfat – while developing tone at the same time. Yes, you will change your overall body shape and improve your health.

But what's even more exciting is the strength you develop, the new-found confidence you'll experience, along with a significant boost in self-esteem and self-worth.

That's why I've titled this book 'Stronger Than Ever'. Those three words encompass everything you can become through weight training: physically strong in the gym, mentally strong outside of it, and simply an overall stronger version of yourself.

And please don't worry that the weight training workouts, or diet advice, will be too difficult. Everything is broken down into plain, understandable language...this is not some sort of scientific journal on nutrition and physiology filled with jargon and complex terminology.

This is not the place for that, there are plenty of sports science books and studies out there on the web if you want to dive deep on all things sports, nutrition and the human body.

Instead, this book is going to show you the way to achievable fitness goals in the gym, and provide practical ways to create weight training workouts and become really confident working out on your own, or with a training partner.

In addition to feeling stronger each time you hit the gym, you should also fully expect feelings of achievement after every workout.

I'm proud of what I've achieved health and fitness wise over the past six years, and I'm about to be upfront and honest with you about that journey, including all the struggles I had to overcome before getting to where I am today. (Even though telling all in a book feels a little scary).

Everything I preach in the upcoming chapters is what I implement in my weekly routine. I'd never recommend or promote something I wasn't fully confident in, or didn't have plenty of experience in.

I want to make you a promise right now. A big promise...

You will absolutely burn bodyfat effectively through weight training, become more toned, settle on an easier, more enjoyable way of eating, and ultimately become a stronger person physically and mentally if you implement what is presented in the upcoming chapters.

There are just three conditions:

#1 Hard work.

#2 Consistency.

#3 Patience.

What are you waiting for? If you're ready to make some serious positive changes in your life through weight training, then let's get started on your journey to become Stronger Than Ever.

Chapter 1

Her Versus Her

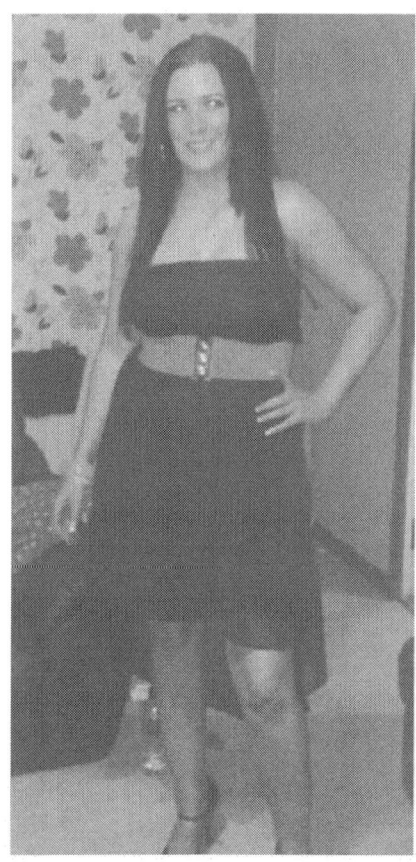
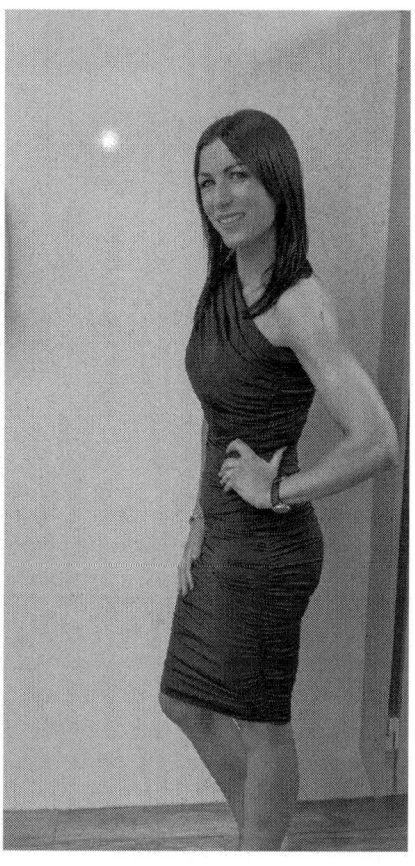

Let's start by introducing two women both into fitness: Miss O and Miss V.

One of these women eats 1,000 calories per day on average, while the other eats double that amount.

One of these women does HIIT workouts out at home, while the other does weight training at the gym.

One of these women is 29 years old. The other is 37 years old.

Have you guessed who is who yet?

Miss O

Miss O on the left is Miss Old Me – a picture that was taken in 2012 when I was aged 29. Back then I weighed 170lbs (12 stones) and realised I had to take some serious action to get back to my natural slimmer shape.

What got me to that stage was poor food choices, lack of exercise for too long, work and studying stresses, and trying to fit everything in while being a mum to a five-year-old girl.

By the time the above photo was taken I had begun doing high intensity cardio workouts at home, jumping about my living room to a DVD routine.

I also cut my calories right down to 1,000 per day max. I mistakenly thought that reducing the amount of food I ate was the only way to shed the weight and get my old body back.

Don't get me wrong, it worked in terms of the numbers on the bathroom scales. The daily calorie restriction did result in me becoming lighter, but there were several downsides.

- I eventually became 'skinny fat' – while I lost some fat, I didn't lose it all and I had virtually no muscle tone. It meant I went from one body shape I didn't like to another I wasn't satisfied with. The extreme calorie restriction + cardio workouts didn't deliver.

- I looked like crap – I'm talking about my skin, my eyes etc. I felt I lacked vitality that I had years previously and wasn't the picture of health I had been before.

- I was physically drained – the constant calorie cutting left me with no energy, and it was a struggle finding the motivation to perform those high intensity workouts at home.

- I was mentally drained – trying to maintain a low-calorie diet and resist all your favourite foods when there's temptation everywhere takes a lot of willpower and it eventually gets to you. It wasn't fun, and if your health and fitness regime isn't fun then it's not going to last. Mine didn't.

Miss V

Miss V on the right is me, Victoria Murphy, in 2019. This photo was taken at a friend's party in December and I'd turned 37 years old the previous month.

Several people who have seen both the pictures above side by side have told me that I look 29 in the picture on the right, not the one on the left. And these days I'm 50lbs lighter.

I put the difference between the old me and the new version of me down to weight training and my sensible, enjoyable way of eating these days.

I don't really get hung up on what age I look, it's not that important. What is important to me is how I feel – and my weight training and nutrition lifestyle makes me feel amazing more often than not.

Here's the difference in terms of how I live my life:

- I don't restrict calories and don't count them either – I put more emphasis on eating unprocessed, whole foods, doing plenty of home cooking, and minimising sugar intake. From past experience, I know that I roughly take in between 1,700 and 2,000 calories each day...much more than before.

- I do intermittent fasting five days per week – which automatically burns fat and keeps me nice and healthy. There has been a lot of positive information released about the huge benefits of intermittent fasting in recent years...to the point where I think everyone should be doing it. This way of eating puts more emphasis on the timing of your meals, rather than focusing solely on what types of foods you're eating. We'll go into more detail on intermittent fasting later.

- I absolutely LOVE my workouts – before it became a struggle when trying to get motivated for the same old cardio workouts. I also never got much satisfaction out of them, instinctively knowing that they were preventing me from gaining lots of weight – but barely changing my body shape. Weight training is completely different, I'm excited about stepping into the gym and pushing myself hard because it produces excellent results.

- I feel so strong physically and mentally – one of the biggest messages I want to get across early in this book is that it's less about the aesthetics and more about the mental benefits that come with lifting weights. By strengthening your body and testing your muscles you'll also be strengthening your mind and developing your self-esteem.

In the upcoming chapters I'm going to describe a series of super effective weight training exercises, and explain how to formulate workout plans that work.

Every time you step out of the gym after these workouts, you'll have grown in confidence and be ready to take on the world.

Chapter 2

Feeling Intimidated In The Gym

"Look at her, she doesn't have a clue what she's doing."

"That girl doesn't belong here, the weights section is for guys."

"What's she doing? That's not how you lift weights."

The criticisms were fierce. They made me feel small. I was a nervous wreck.

I heard those harsh words over and over. How could I ever hope to give up boring cardio and lift weights in the gym when these types of judgements were thrown my way?

How dare an unfit, out-of-shape mum like me even step into the weights section among all these men with criticisms like this?

And here's the worst part: those criticisms were coming from ME.

Yep, the voice in my head was creating all this noise. No-one in the gym had said a single negative word to me about my desire to lift weights.

Not the guy with huge arms doing bicep curls, not the sweaty dude with the Beats headphones on, and not the teenage lads messing about with their mobile phones next to the dumbbell rack.

But that irritating voice in my head had plenty to say. She was loud, repetitive, and had basically created a brick wall of fear for me. Yet again.

I had always managed to maintain my poker face in the gym, but those familiar waves of nervousness kept crashing around in my stomach for every second I even looked in the direction of the weights section.

What did I do that day? I did what I'd done for the previous five months...

I strolled over to the long row of treadmills and joined a long line of people either jogging or walking briskly on the spot. They were getting nowhere – literally. Neither was I.

It was December 2014 and I was essentially paying £30 per month for a gym membership to walk and jog. Why was I bothering? I could have done the same outside in the fresh air for free.

I'd been a member of my local gym for five months and I'm surprised I even lasted that long because I was doing the same old boring routine. Fifteen minutes on the treadmill, five minutes on the rowing machine, 10 minutes on the exercise bike, and rounding it off with some abs exercises on the mat on the floor.

I always worked my ass off; determined to get back to the shape I was in before my daughter was born. And no matter how boring all the cardio training was, I didn't skip any of the exercises or leave early.

Yet no matter how many times I looked in the mirror when I got home from the gym I saw zero changes in my body shape. And I tried looking from every angle possible.

I can't remember how I discovered that weight training was the answer to achieving my fitness goals. I don't know when exactly the penny dropped.

All I know is that I felt insecure about lifting weights in the gym, and felt intimidated by the idea of mingling in that part of the gym that was populated by guys.

I tried to persuade some of my girl friends to train with me. Safety in numbers, and all that. But they weren't interested – they didn't want to get "too bulky".

It was just me vs my fears...and I had seven of them.

My 7 Weightlifting Worries

#1 Attempting an exercise and not being able to do it (#humiliation).

#2 People laughing at me (#morehumiliation).

#3 Forgetting my workout routine.

#4 Looking stupid doing every exercise – and feeling stupider for even attempting them. (And yes, sometimes I make words up).

#5 Pulling silly faces looking like I'm constipated - or making random grunting noises.

#6 Dropping a weight on my foot — or some other poor victim's foot.

#7 Tripping up, falling into a stranger, causing them to bang into another stranger...and wrecking everyone's day.

****

I know for certain that many women feel the exact same when it comes to weight training. The same insecurities rise to the surface and we fear we'll be judged on how we look, and how well we perform each of these exercises that are new to us.

The reason I know is that every single woman I've spoken to who does strength training, or used to lift weights in the past, has told me so.

Once you quickly get past the scary, awkward stage, it becomes okay to openly admit you were terrified the first time you picked up a dumbbell in public.

But how do you get to that stage? How did I finally build up the courage after five months to leave the cardio equipment behind and march boldly into the weights area for a proper workout?

Below I've listed 5 key steps that will ensure you can build up enough confidence and motivation to hit the weights, and start transforming your body quicker than ever before.

5 Steps To Confidence In The Gym

#1 Always go light at first

When you first start weight training, simply go nice and light in the beginning. Get familiar with the dumbbells and barbells, and focus only on mastering your exercise technique.

Correct technique should always come first, you can increase the weight further down the line when you're more experienced.

By taking the lighter approach, it also means there's virtually zero chance of any of those nightmare scenarios in your head ever materialising. You know the ones. I'm talking about our fears of dropping heavy dumbbells, squatting and not being able to get back up again, or slipping with a barbell above your head.

#2 Get clued up on each exercise before you physically do them

Do your research on all weight training exercises before you even attempt them. Look at pictures, watch videos...and keep reading this book.

In the upcoming chapters I'm going to go in-depth on 26 highly-effective exercises you should be including in your weight training workouts – in order to get the best results.

These include my 13 top essential exercises you should do regularly in the gym, and a further 13 exercises that I incorporate frequently into sessions for variety and to keep working the muscles hard.

I've included photos of me performing every move, along with clear instructions on what to do and what to avoid. This will definitely help boost your confidence for when you put it all into practice.

#3 Find a training partner

Remember, you're not alone. The vast majority of women have hang-ups about getting started with weight training. So why not ask a friend who is also looking to get fit and improve her body shape to be your training partner?

When you've got someone close you can chat to and have a laugh with, it'll help you relax in the gym and worry less about what other people think.

You and your gym buddy can push each other on, which will obviously improve your gym performance too. There's also much less chance of you lying on the sofa instead of going to the gym when you know that someone else is expecting to work out with you.

#4 Go to the gym at an off-peak time

In every gym I've ever gone to, I've discovered that they're busiest at three main stages of the day (Monday-Friday):

- 7am-8.30am: generally busy professionals looking to squeeze in a gym session before work, aswell as some early risers.
- 12noon-1pm: people who have flocked to the gym on their work lunch break.
- 5pm-8pm: the rush of people heading to the gym after their 9-5 jobs.

So, you can see that there are opportunities to slip into the gym when it's not busy and, if you're lucky, you might even have the weights section to yourself for 30-60 mins.

Arriving at the gym at an-off peak time is exactly what I did when I finally built up the courage to do my first weight training workout. I turned up at 2pm on a Tuesday, and there was one older man at the weights section...and probably five people in the entire gym.

#5 Get in your discomfort zone

All of the previous four steps will undoubtedly boost your confidence levels and by preparing in these ways you'll be ready to go for it in the gym.

But even if you're still a bit nervous and insecure about the prospect, remember that strength comes from putting yourself in uncomfortable situations and coming through them.

Get in your discomfort zone. You'll feel amazing afterwards.

It's All About You

I'll be honest, the gym fear and nervousness didn't magically go away after that first weight training session. It took a couple of months before I was completely comfortable in that public environment, just as I'd be in a supermarket or stepping onto a bus.

But every time I went to the gym and picked up a dumbbell the anxiety lessened. Every set of a particular exercise became more natural with less stress and tension. With every workout my confidence grew bit by bit.

Best of all: I began to feel physically stronger, which was something I'd never experienced after years of trying fitness classes, home workout DVDs, and countless other useless training methods.

If you're someone lacking in confidence about weight training, please remember that most people are too self-absorbed in their own world at the gym to even pay you any attention.

I used to think people were judging my workouts and laughing about me, but over time I noticed that people in the gym aren't laughing at you or staring at you.

They're more focused on their own training and reaching their own goals, just like you and I.

It's time for you to focus on you. It's all about you...and the confidence will come; I promise you it will.

It will come with more self-love and acceptance, and pushing yourself physically in the gym to achieve what you haven't done before.

Lifting weights not only strengthens you from a physical level, but it makes you a much stronger, more resilient person overall.

Time to become Stronger Than Ever.

Chapter 3

Lean Not Bulky

Damn it, they must be right!

We were warned that lifting weights would make us big and bulky.

We were worried that we'd end up with muscular arms like men.

We never listened to that voice in our head telling us that it would be safer to stick with cardio...'just incase' we started to resemble the Incredible Hulk on his rest day from the gym.

And guess what? I finally seen her...the big, bad, bulky weightlifting woman they were all talking about. Huge back, chunk shoulders, and muscular arms. The kind of physique I was worried I'd develop when I switched from cardio to weight training.

Here's the thing: I first spotted this woman doing lifting weights in late November 2019. In five years of me hitting the gym - doing 758 (approximately) weight training workouts – she was the ONLY woman I'd seen that was big and bulky during that time.

She was the exception and it seemed pretty obvious why. She trained like a powerlifter, using chalk, weight belts etc, and undoubtedly followed a bodybuilder-style approach to training and diet.

I'm talking about huge amounts of calories, protein, and adding all sorts of supplements to her weekly regimen to make maximum muscle gains. There may even have been sports enhancers (translation: steroids) added into the mix. Yep, some women do that too, believe it or not.

Now obviously I don't know this woman and don't know everything she does training and nutrition wise to give a full, detailed explanation. I'm also not judging her approach as it takes a lot of gym and nutrition dedication, which I respect, to achieve her specific fitness goals.

My first point is: her results are absolutely not typical.

My second point: you don't need to worry about getting big and bulky through weight training.

The reality is that by lifting weights, increasing the resistance on your muscles, and developing your overall body strength, you can burn fat so much more effectively than cardio – and develop great muscle tone.

And not only can you get in the best shape of your life by leaving boring cardio behind and focusing mainly on weight training, I'm certain you'll enjoy the workouts more and love the physical and mental strength they deliver.

3 Reasons Why You Don't Need To Have The 'Bulky' Fear

#1 Hormones – women simply don't have the same capability of building muscle mass like men. It's the way nature made us. Testosterone is the primary muscle building hormone, and men produce roughly 15 times more of this anabolic hormone than us women.

I'm sure you know that it goes back to the good old days when men killed wildebeest and women stayed in the cave making it all homely. You get the gist.

I'm not suggesting women are weak and men are strong, we just have a different hormonal make-up. Sure, you could eat a tonne of calories and do an intense amount of training, but it's still not going to achieve the same type of muscle growth as men doing the same.

#2 Training frequency – you're not going to be training 5,6,7 days per week with the methods described in this book. You're not an athlete powerlifter.

In order to gain muscle mass, you need to repeatedly put your muscles under tension and couple this with specific dietary protocols.

That's great for elite athletes and bodybuilders who have the time, money, and desire to achieve muscle mass goals.

But if you're a busy mum like me, if you have a full-time job, and just want to get in great shape and stay healthy, you only have to train about four times per week, with no more than one hour per session.

#3 Dietary difference - you're not a bodybuilder that requires wolfing down crazy amounts of calories, protein, and getting all mathematical about grams of carbs.

Athletes, powerlifters, bodybuilders etc have certain targets to reach when it comes to strength, muscle mass, body fat percentages etc. So they either need to eat a huge amount of calories for bulking up, or switch to strict calorie deficits around competition time.

While dietary choices are important when it comes to developing lean muscle and achieving fat loss, I don't get uptight about counting the amounts of carbs, fats and protein (or macros as the cool kids call it). Neither should you.

I just make sure I include good sources of protein, carbs and fat in every meal. And instead of scrimping on calories, I also eat a decent amount of them (food yaaay) to support my body's needs. More to come on that later.

****

I believe now that women are starting to realise the effectiveness of lifting weights for fat loss. It's clear to see in gyms these days. When I first started lifting weights in my local gym five years ago, I was often the only woman at that section.

These days, I see far more women picking up dumbbells and barbells. I also see a big difference in the faces of women in the gym. More often than not, those doing cardio on the treadmills, rowing machine, and exercise bikes look like they're having zero fun – or are pretty much bored out of their skulls.

Whereas in the weights section, you see looks of determination and a few more smiles. It's more fun when you're testing yourself with heavier weights, and realise you're stronger than you thought you were. It builds your confidence.

I used to think the women in the best shape must do more cardio than me and eat fewer calories than me. The reality is the opposite. Those with the lean muscle, toned arms and legs, and no jiggly bits are those who learned quickly that weight training is the way to go.

I respect all forms of training and goal setting when it comes to health and fitness. Everyone is on their own journey whether it be fat loss, muscle gain, fitness modelling, powerlifting or sumo wrestling.

The approach I have is to develop a strong, healthy body as I believe it develops a strong, healthy mind. I've seen countless other women just like you achieve the same.

My journey through weight training has helped me develop confidence, self-love, and self-acceptance, and helped me grow both on a personal and professional level. The progress you make in the gym somehow carries on outside of it too.

I remember when I used to loathe my body and dream of being in amazing shape, but strength training has changed my thought process and belief system.

My view is not to hate my body when it has a bit of fat, or maybe some cellulite, or stress over every tiny imperfection. Weight training has given me mental strength to accept the imperfections and love my body the way it is.

I don't know you, but I know it can do the same for you.

WEIGHT TRAINING EXERCISES
··
THE 13
FUNDAMENTALS

CHAPTER 4

Warming Up For The 13 Fundamentals

In the upcoming pages I'm going to share descriptions and picture demonstrations of me doing my top 13 exercises, which I consider weight training fundamentals for women.

These are exercises I've found to be most effective and do regularly in the gym. Not only do I think they're the best, but I get the most fun out of doing them.

I'd like to thank Jamal and the team at Energie Fitness in Dumbarton, my local gym, for allowing me to take the upcoming pictures at their premises. It's a fantastic gym and you can check out their Facebook page here:

www.facebook.com/EnergieFitnessD

Then in the next chapter we'll cover another 13 great exercises to add into the mix that will help work your body hard and add variation to your weight training workouts.

But before all the weightlifting action begins, I've got to stress the importance of two things:

- Warming up well first before lifting weights.
- Correct exercise technique on every exercise, every time.

A typical warm-up should take around five minutes and involve lots of stretches for your legs and arms; yoga stretches are very beneficial.

And with any weightlifting exercises you're not familiar with, try practicing the move first before adding any weight to it. For example, do the upright row with the bar only and no weighted discs on either side until you feel comfortable with the move.

Correct exercise form is so important when weight training, otherwise you could be setting yourself up for injury.

If you don't feel comfortable practicing form in the gym, then do so at home in front of the mirror, or even record a video of yourself to make sure it looks and feels safe.

Okay, let's begin with an exercise that'll do wonders for your legs, bum, and core...squats.

BARBELL SQUATS

It's time to hit the lower body muscles hard with the mighty barbell squats.

Muscles worked

Quadriceps, hamstrings, glutes, calves, core, lower back.

What to do

1. Place a barbell on a squat rack at shoulder height or slightly below.

2. Add weights discs to either side of the bar (one each side at a time) and lock them in place with safety collars. (* Note, an Olympic barbell weighs 20kg alone).

3. Duck your head underneath the bar and bring your upper back and hands up until the barbell is resting on your shoulder blades.

4. Push upwards with your legs so that your back lifts the barbell off the rack, and then take 2 small steps backwards away from the squat rack.

5. Stand upright with your feet at hip width, your back straight, and looking directly ahead in the mirror.

6. Squat downwards with the weight, keeping your upper body and core rigid, allowing your legs to do the work bringing you down.

7. Once your legs reach a 90 degree angle (i.e. your thighs are parallel with the floor), then push back up forcefully to the starting position, again keeping your back and core firm.

** Note: some women can squat lower to the ground, some can't quite reach that 90 degree angle I describe. Our bodies are all different shapes and sizes, so there's no wrong answer. Just try to get as close to the 90 degree angle as possible.

What NOT to do

1. Don't forget to lock the weight discs in place at the end of the bar. They could fall off otherwise during the exercise.

2. As always, don't look down at the floor. Keep your gaze focused straight ahead throughout every single repetition.

3. Don't move your feet during the exercise as this could throw you off balance. Keep them planted in the same spot throughout your repetitions.

4. I've mentioned this at the beginning of this chapter, but this is just a friendly reminder: always lift lighter at first when doing exercises like these. You can start increasing the weight once you're comfortable with the technique.

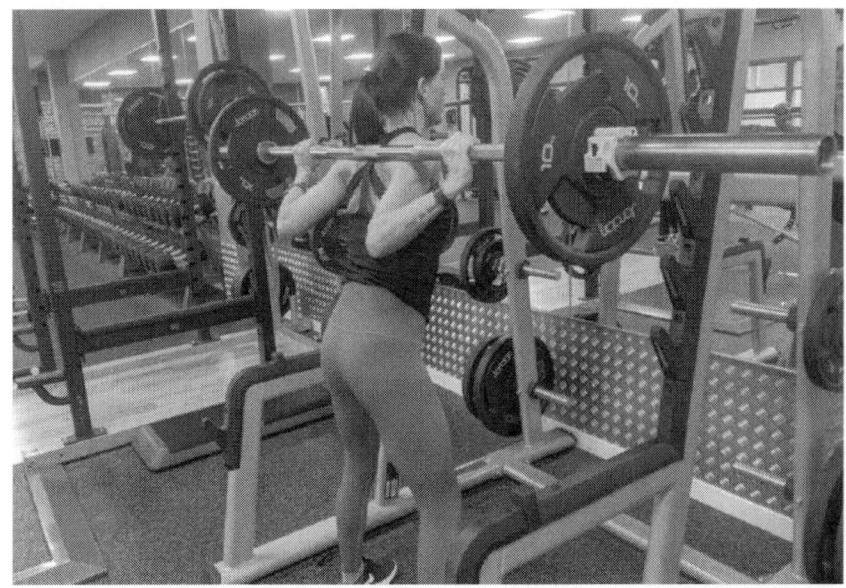

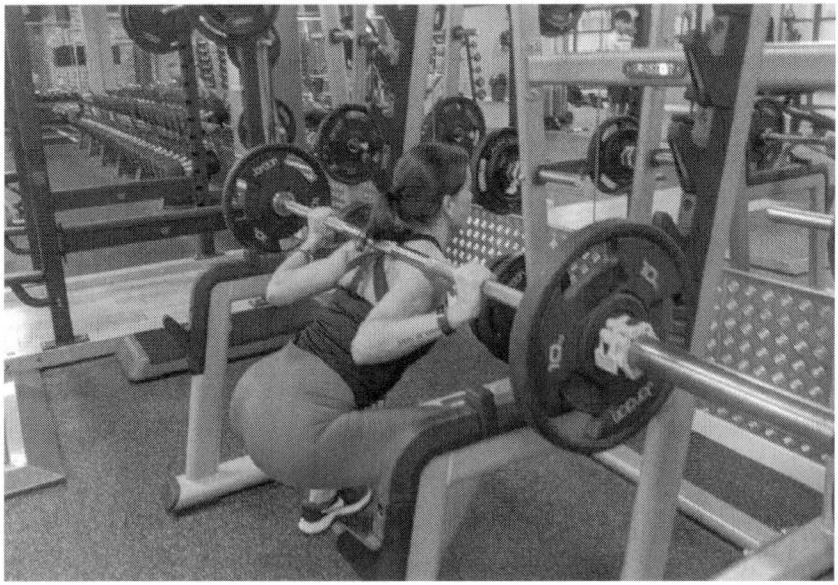

HIP THRUSTS

I think this is at the top of the list when it comes to building a strong and solid set of glutes.

Again, technique is so important for this exercise, so I suggest practicing this without a weight either in the gym or at home first.

Muscles worked

Glutes, hamstrings.

What to do

1. Find a bench and a barbell. Sitting on the floor, place the barbell across the top of your thighs – you can use a pad or towel to stop it from digging in.

2. Next step is to rest your back across the bench, I like to have the side of the bench cushion just at the base of my shoulders.

3. Your feet should be placed directly under your knees, hip width apart, so that when you fully extend into the movement, your legs make a 90 degree angle.

4. Place your hands on top of the bar. Lift the bar with your hips in a driving upwards motion, while engaging your core and glutes during the entire exercise. Keep a straight back once at the top of the movement, don't over-arch your back.

5. While doing this, I like to pretend to have an egg under my chin and that I'm trying to hold it there. If you look up the egg will fall and if you push you chin down, you'll break the egg. That's the ideal position you want.

6. If you feel this movement is working your quads or back, try to re-adjust your feet. This is an exercise that targets your glutes and you'll know when it feels right.

7. Once you have the hang of this you can add weights – it shouldn't take long. The glutes are one of the strongest muscle groups in the human body and can easily cope with a heavy weight.

What NOT to do

1. Hyper-extend the lower back.

2. Have your feet too far away or too close to your body.

3. Push up onto toes.

4. Have your back too far across or too far off the bench.

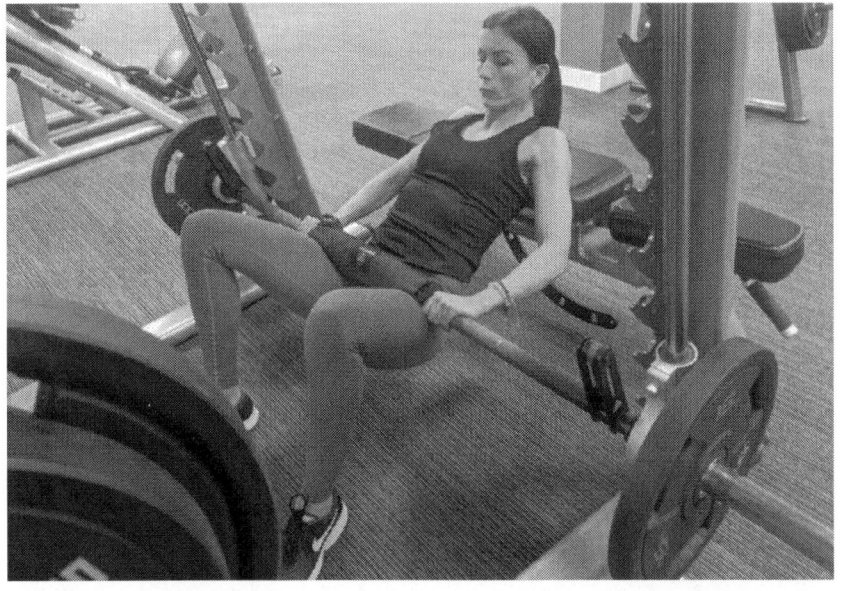

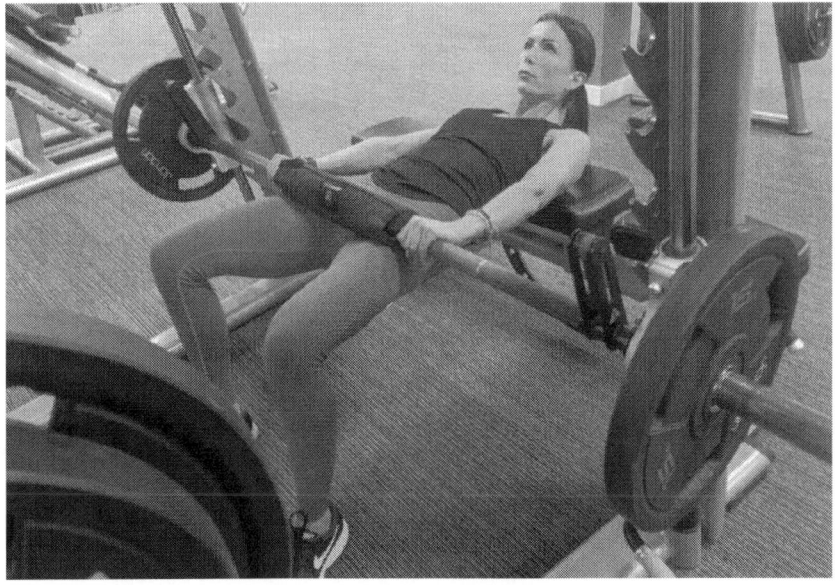

CHIN-UPS

I know what most readers are thinking: "I'll never be able to do chin-ups!"

That's exactly what I thought too when I first started out in the gym. Sure, it's a very tough exercise, but please don't be put off by that.

If you follow my advice and train consistently, you'll gradually build up enough strength and eventually be able to smash chin-ups out like a pro. Trust me.

At first I started off at home with a bar on a door frame, then an assisted machine in the gym, and resistance bands. Eventually I was finally able to do one unassisted rep – and there's no better feeling!

I'm going to describe two methods that'll help you master the exercise technique, gradually develop your upper body strength, and then progress towards doing proper unassisted reps.

This could take weeks, it could take months, but by following these steps you'll absolutely make steady progress. And as this exercise works several muscles groups at once, you'll tone your upper body very nicely along the way.

Muscles worked

Shoulder, biceps, lats, forearms, core.

Method 1: Using an assistance machine

These machines are designed to support some of your bodyweight while you do the exercise, and essentially gives you a helping hand.

As you get stronger week by week, you gradually lower the weight assistance on the machine. This means it supports less of your bodyweight and thus moves closer towards you proper reps.

Once you can do 10-12 reps with good technique at the lowest support level on the machine, you'll then be ready to attempt your first chin-up.

What to do

1. Set the pin on the assistance machine to a suitable level to support your bodyweight. If you have a lot of weight to lose, then I'd suggest putting the pin at one of the highest levels at the beginning.

2. Stand on the support lever and reach up grabbing the chin-up handles above with an underhand grip (i.e. your palms facing you).

* Note: some assisted machines have a square cushion rather than a lever in the next pictures. If that's the case, then rest your knees on the cushion for support.

Also, if the chin-up handles point out the way, then simply grab them with your palms facing inward towards each other.

3. Pull yourself up to the top of the machine, with your chin in line with or slightly above the handles, then lower yourself until your arms are almost straight but not completely locked out at the elbow.

4. Pull yourself back up again forcefully, squeezing your arms until you reach the top of machine again. Then repeat.

What NOT to do

1. Don't perform 'half reps'. By this I mean, only dropping your body halfway and not extending your arms enough. This doesn't work the muscles properly.

2. Don't give up because chin-ups seem too difficult at first. You'll get there. Perseverance pays off.

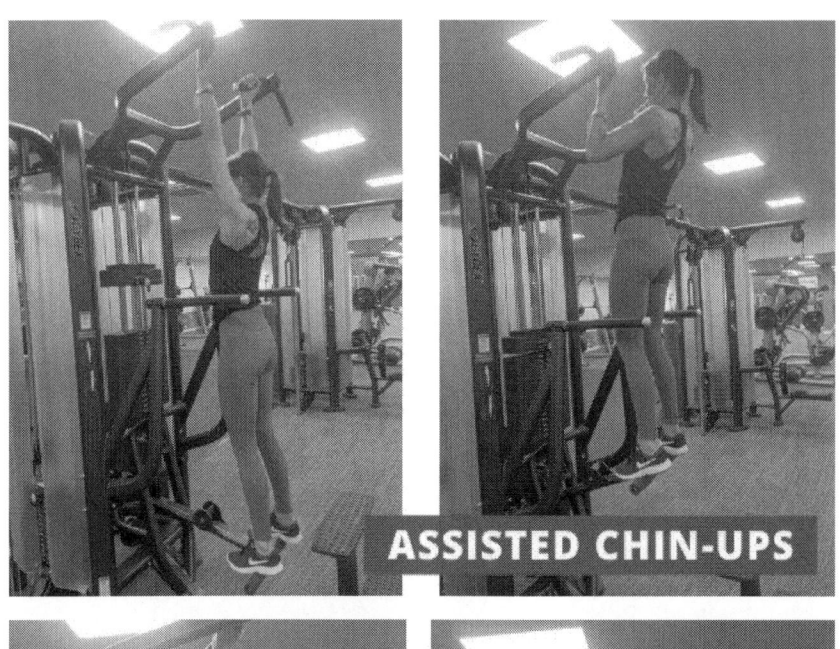

ASSISTED CHIN-UPS

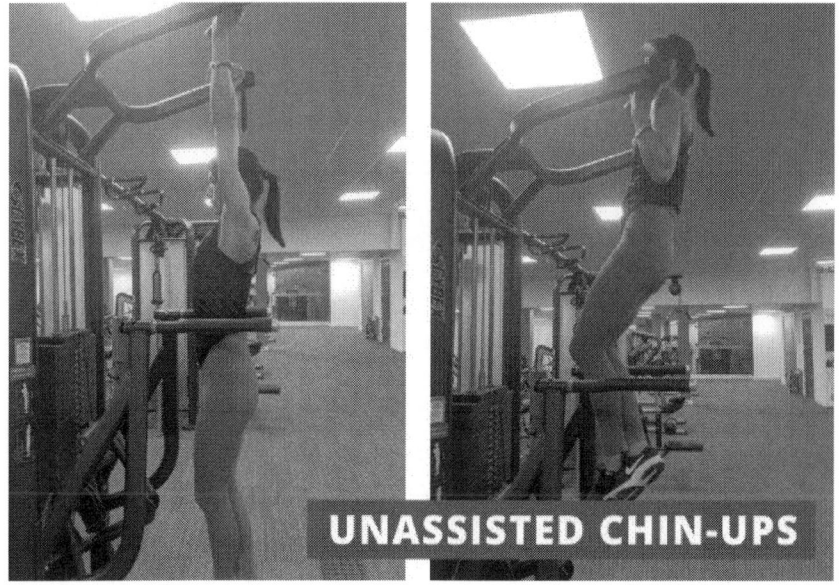

UNASSISTED CHIN-UPS

DIPS

This is another fantastic upper body exercise for toning your arms, shoulders, and developing upper body strength.

As it's a bodyweight exercise, just like chin-ups, most people require support using an assistance machine or resistance bands. We'll cover both on the next couple of pages.

Muscles worked

Triceps, chest, shoulders, forearms, core.

Method 1: Using an assistance machine.

What to do

1. Set the pin to a suitable weights level on the machine; enough to support your weight when you're doing the exercise. You may have to experiment a little to find the ideal level.

2. Step up to the lever, and stand on it while grabbing onto the dip bar handles with each hand. Your palms should be facing inwards towards each other.

3. Hold your body upright with your arms straight, and look straight ahead.

4. Then bend your elbows and lower your body until your arms are at a 90 degree angle.

5. Push back upwards, extending your arms all way until they are straight and lock out at the elbow again.

6. Repeat as many reps as possible, always maintaining good technique.

What NOT to do

1. Don't lean forward during the exercise, try to keep your back fairly upright as you move up and down.

2. Don't look down towards the floor as doing this tends to result in leaning forward and ruining the exercise technique. Always look straight ahead and stay focused.

3. As always, don't perform half reps by only bending the elbows slightly. Make sure you come down low enough so that your arms are roughly at a 90 degree angle.

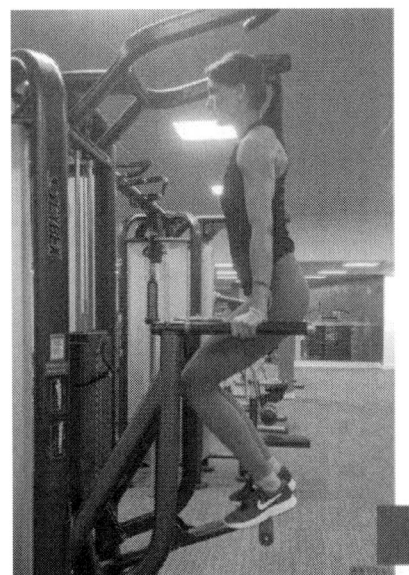
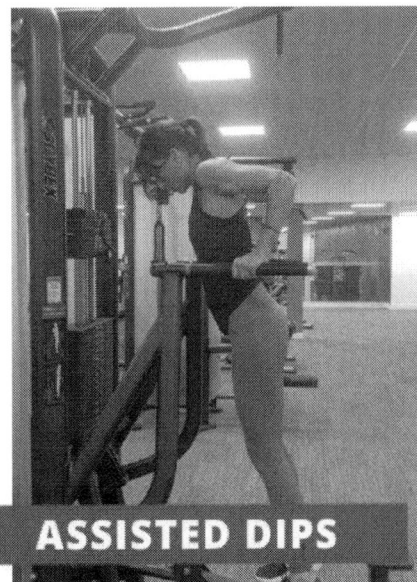

ASSISTED DIPS

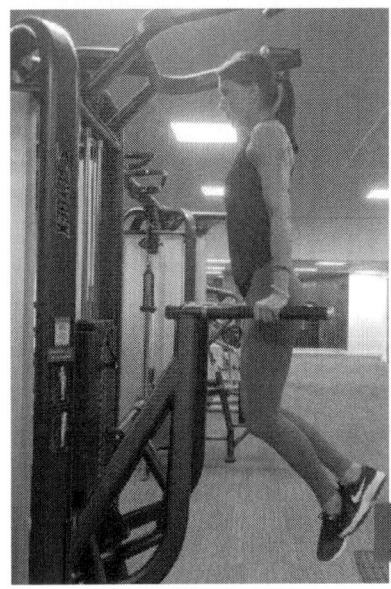
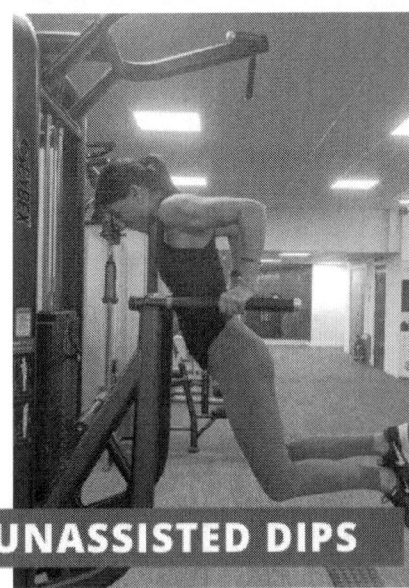

UNASSISTED DIPS

BENCH PRESS

The bench press is the well-known gym exercise where you're lying on a bench with your feet on the floor pressing a barbell with weights up and down.

It's a really good exercise for toning your shoulders and arms. While it's a little tricky at first, this description below will help you get up to speed in no time.

Muscles worked

Chest, shoulders, triceps.

What to do

1. Find a bench press station (flat bench with rack and barbell sitting on it overhead) and always make sure the weights on each side are not too heavy. Then check that the weights discs are locked in place with safety collars.

(* If you're a complete beginner then start with the bar only because they generally weigh 15-20kg on their own).

2. Lie back on the bench and get in the right position by making sure your eyes are in line with the bar above.

3. Grab the bar with your palms facing upwards, and with your hands at slightly wider than shoulder width.

4. Lift the barbell up off the rack and then bring it forward slightly so that it moves in line with your chest.

5. With your arms straight, steady yourself for a second until you feel in a comfortable position. Then bend your arms and lower the bar in a controlled fashion.

6. When the bar reaches your chest area, press back up forcefully until your arms are straight again. Then repeat until you reach your maximum number of reps in that particular set.

What NOT to do

1. Never begin before double checking the amount of weight loaded onto each side of the bar – it's not much fun ending up pinned to a bench!

2. Don't forget to latch the safety collars onto each end of the bar. Otherwise the weights could slip off each side.

3. Don't raise your lower back off the bench. This is a common mistake people make when lifting heavier than they should...and it's an injury waiting to happen.

4. Don't 'drop' the bar too quickly in the first part of the move. While you shouldn't be lowering the bar too slowly either, it's important that you're in control of the weight when bringing it down to your chest.

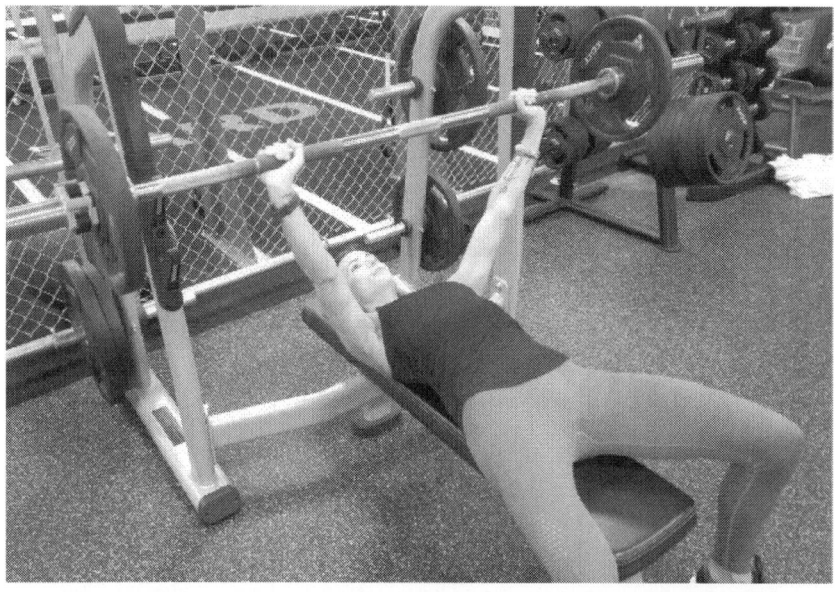

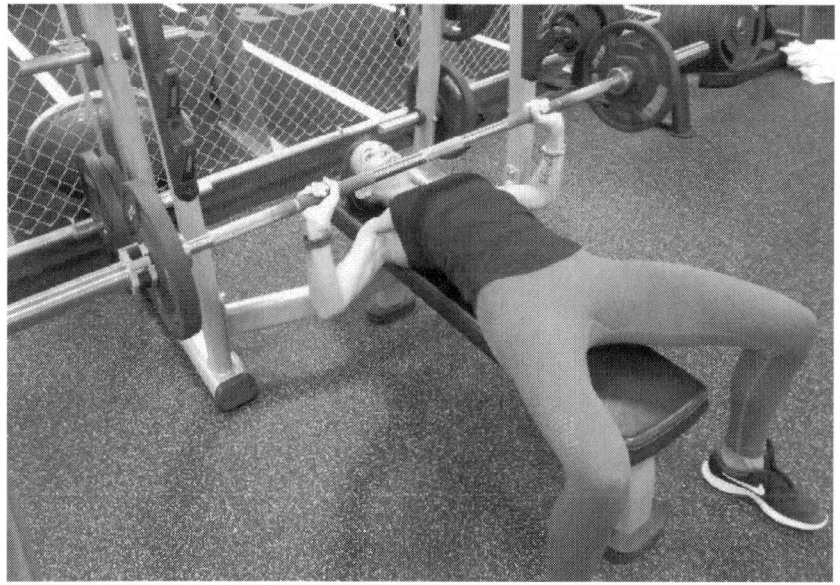

BENT OVER ROW (underhand grip)

Not only is this one of my top exercises but it helps assist in other exercises by allowing you to practice proper hip hinge movements.

Muscles worked

Lats, core, shoulders, trapezius, biceps, forearms, and it also indirectly works hamstring and glutes.

What to do

1. Grab a barbell (bearing in mind these weigh 15-20kg) with an underhand grip, just outside shoulder width apart. Feel free to add disc weights to each side.

2. Hinge forward and push your hips back, while engaging your core and retracting your shoulders back slightly. You want to aim for the bar to be slightly below your knees, while having your lower back flat, no slouching.

3. Move your elbows back, keeping them close to your body, bringing the bar close to your abdomen. Pushing your chest out while pulling the bar back.

4. Squeeze for muscular contraction and then slowly lower the bar to the starting point.

5. Repeat 9-12 times before safely lowering to the floor.

What NOT to do

1. Pulling your body towards the bar. Let your muscles lift and support the weight. Holding a solid, engaged frame is so important while working the targeted muscles.

2. Pull the elbows too far back. Yeah that squeeze at the back may feel good but it can put the shoulder under tremendous strain and after time may cause serious injury. You want the movement to feel natural.

3. Move elbows out to the side. This could again cause a whole host of injuries. You want to stay as engaged as possible.

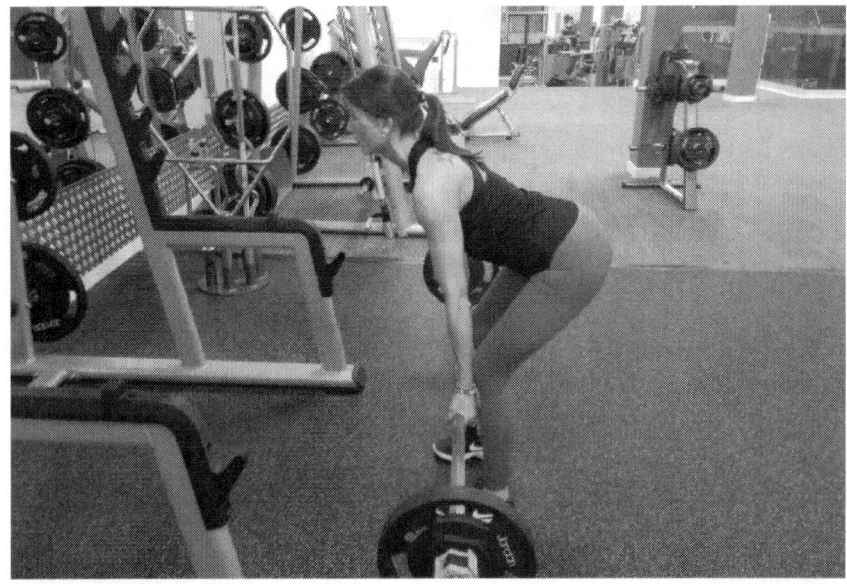

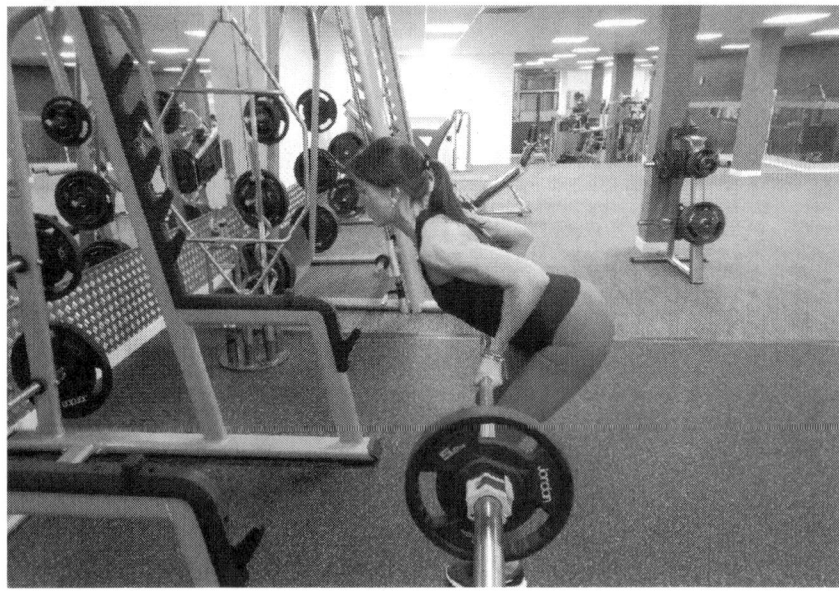

LEG PRESS

I took me a while to incorporate this into my routine. I would always use free weights as I thought they were the best in terms of developing muscle tone.

About a year ago, a friend had mentioned using the leg press machine in the gym and how, if used correctly, can help develop hamstrings and glutes.

So, I started using it at the beginning of my workouts to fire up my glutes and hamstrings before tackling the free weight.

Since then, I've noticed a massive difference and my leg strength and ability overall.

Muscles worked

Glutes, hamstrings, quads, inner thighs, calves.

What to do

1. Initially, don't add any weight as the leg press machines as they generally already have a starting weight, so it's ideal to do a warm-up set with that first.

2. Sit on the seat and place your feet high up on the press plate, a bit wider than hip width, toes pointing forward. There's usually a little safety catch on the machine that you can adjust for depth.

3. Push your feet forward and release the safety bars at the same time – most leg press have them, they're usually at each side of the seat, where your hands will rest.

4. Allow the plate to lower towards you while keeping your back straight and core engaged. You should feel the tension on the hamstrings and glutes.

5. Push back to starting position with your heels but don't lock out the knees, keep a slight bend when extending.

What NOT to do

1. Load with heavy weights before trying it out first.

2. Push the plate back with your toes, hands etc.

3. Lean forward – back straight and core engaged at all times.

4. Allow your knees to fall inwards – again this will put the knee in a compromising position, you want the movement to be natural. If you find your knees going inward them aim to push them out when pushing the plate back up or aim for a lighter weight until you have the technique mastered.

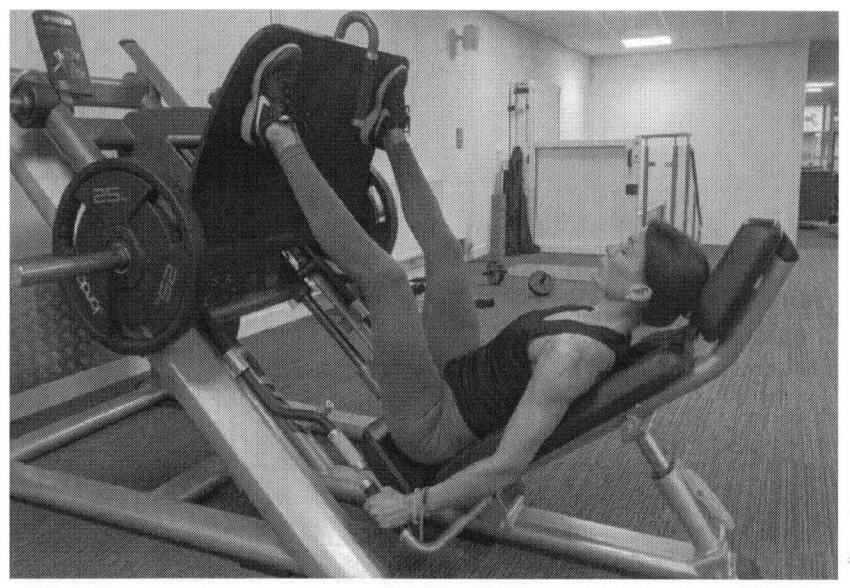

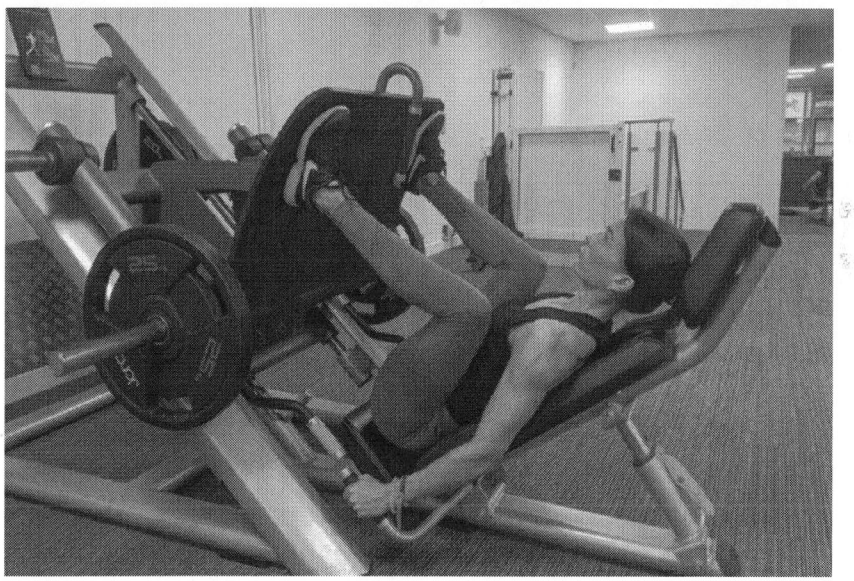

LANDMINE SQUATS

I love squat variations. I quickly got a bit fed up with using the back squat routinely so after some research I found this little beauty and use it regularly, I think it really helps in developing the leg muscles.

Muscles worked

Quadriceps, glutes, hamstrings, calves.

What to do

1. Insert bar into a landmine unit if your gym has one or wedge it into a corner.

2. Pick up the other end of the bar and hold it about 10cm from your chest.

3. Adjust feet a bit wider than shoulder width, toes pointing at a slight angle outward.

4. Push your hips back and perform the squat the same as before in the previous exercise. Keep your spine neutral, core engaged and shoulders slightly back. Aim to go as deep as possible.

5. Push back up to the starting position through your heels.

6. Once you become comfortable with this movement, you can aim to push the bar up above your head while rising up from the squat, this will add more muscles worked to the exercise. Such as the lats and shoulders. Feel comfortable with the initial squats first though.

What NOT to do

1. Hold the bar close to your chest.

2. Lean forward – this will compromise your lower back and shoulder and could set you up for injury.

3. Take the weight on your toes – this will put strain on your knees.

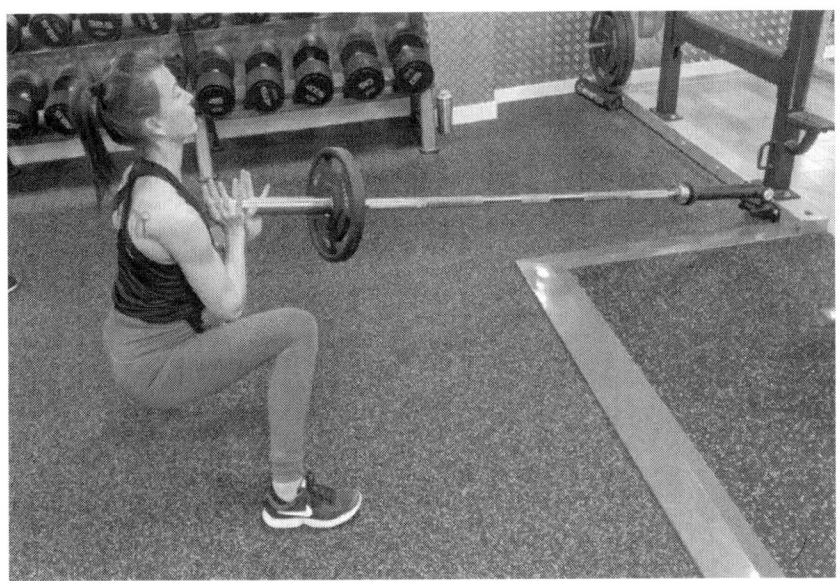

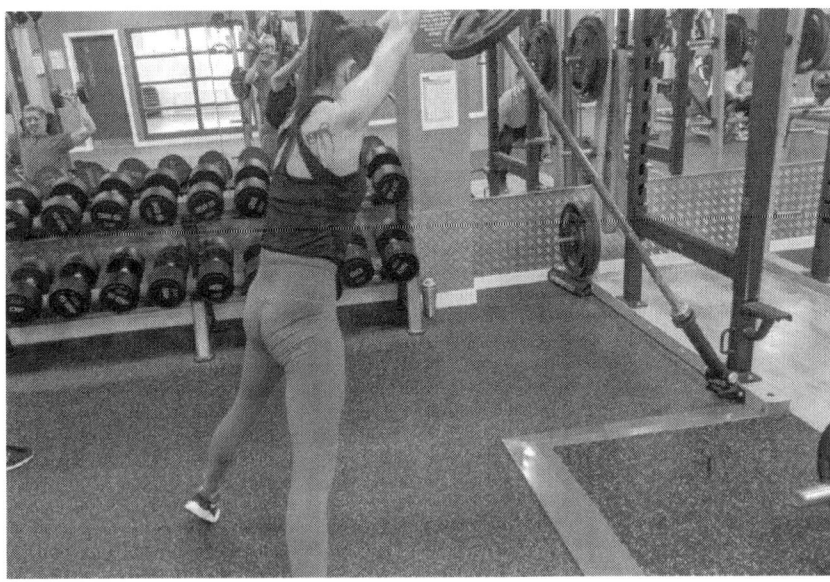

STRAIGHT LEG DEADLIFT

I loooove this move. I naturally build muscle to the front part of my legs and used to find it quite difficult build strong hamstrings and glutes.

This exercise took my training to a whole new level. You can feel the burn in your hamstrings from the get-go.

Muscles worked

Hamstrings, glutes, lower back, lats.

What to do

1. Stand straight with feet hip width apart, toes pointing forward or slightly out.

2. Just like the bent over row, hold the barbell but this time have an overhand grip, a bit wider than shoulder width, in front of your thighs.

Don't lock out the knees, keep a slight bend in them. And, as always, keep your shoulders back and don't slouch.

3. As before, drive the hips back while keeping your shoulders back and chest forward, while lowering the bar to your shins. You should feel the hamstring reach full stretch, don't round your back, neutral spine always.

4. Pull the bar back to the start of the move by using your hamstrings, engage the glutes when your reach the top of the movement, don't lock out your knees.

What NOT to do

1. Don't jerk, twist or bounce during the movement.

2. Keep a neutral spine, never look too far up or too far down, this puts your spine in a compromising position

3. The bar should go straight up and down, keeping close to the body. Don't allow the bar to move out away from you.

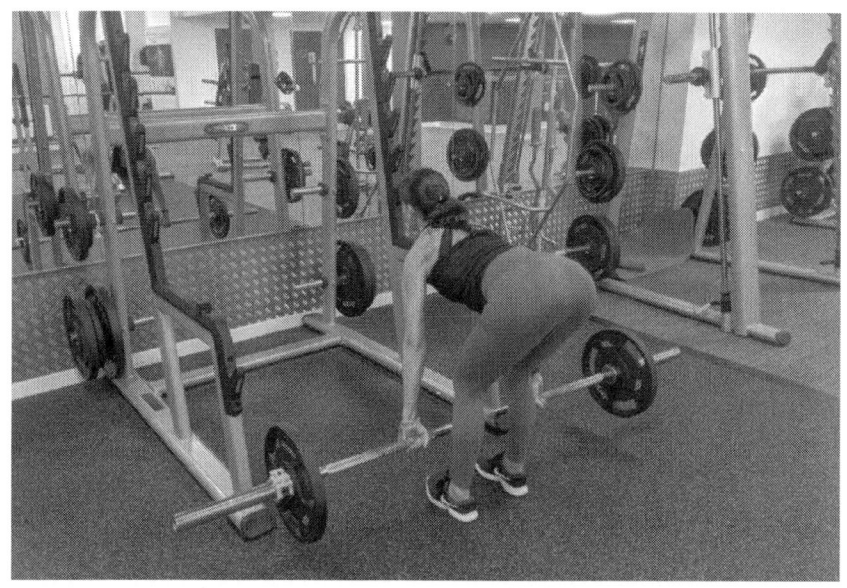

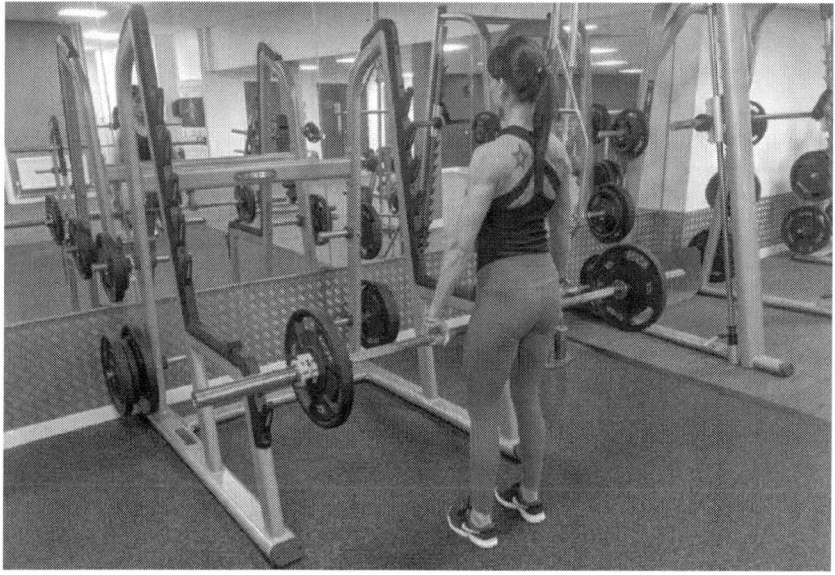

TRICEPS KICKBACK

This exercise is a good isolation movement. I like to incorporate it with other upper body exercises.

You can totally feel the burn with this...

Muscles worked

Triceps, forearms.

What to do

1. Grab a couple of dumbbells and hold them by your side.

2. Engage your core and keep a neutral spine. Hinge forward at the waist, pushing your hips back and bringing your torso almost parallel to the floor.

3. Aim to keep your arms in close to your body and your head in line with your spine, tuck your chin in slightly – like holding the egg again.

4. Engage your triceps by straightening your elbows. Move only your forearms during this movement, keep your upper arms still.

5. Pause here for a second before returning the weights to the starting position.

What NOT to do

1. Jerk or bounce during the movement, the only thing that should be moving should be your forearms.

2. Over arch your spine.

3. Go too heavy, this exercise can be tricky to master and you don't want to compromise the integrity of the shoulders by trying to move a weight too heavy.

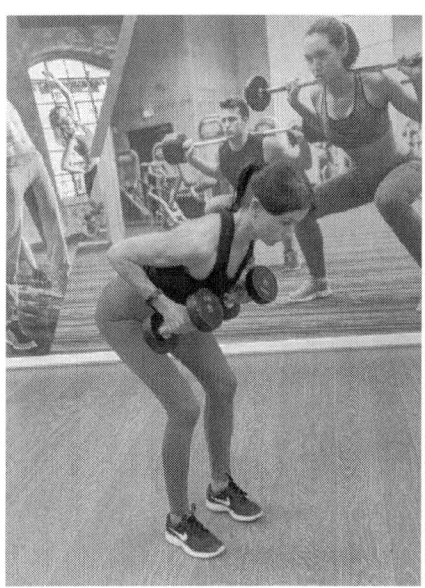
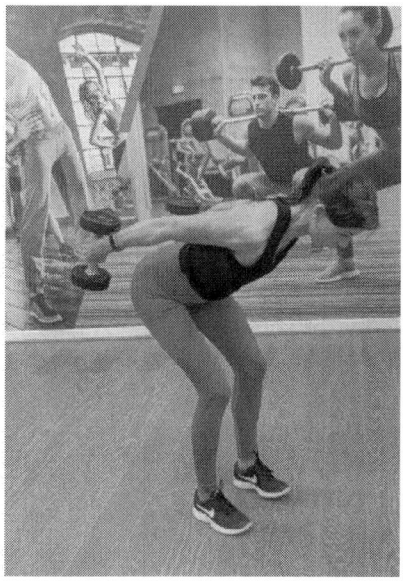

REVERSE FLYES

This is one of my favourite exercises for working the back and shoulders. It's a pretty straightforward dumbbells move that you'll be able to master quickly.

Muscles worked

Lats, trapezius, rear area of shoulders.

What to do

1. Grab two dumbbells of the same weight from the rack, and stand in front of a mirror.

2. With your feet slightly apart and knees slightly bent, lean forward with your arms hanging down with a dumbbell in each hand facing (palms facing inwards - as shown in the following pictures).

3. While looking straight ahead, raise your arms up in a 'flying' motion with the dumbbells in your hands.

4. Once your arms are parallel with the floor, lower the dumbbells again in a controlled manner until they meet again in front of your thighs.

5. Repeat until your complete a full set of repetitions.

What NOT to do

1. As always don't look downwards at the floor as this will affect your posture. Keep your gaze on yourself in the mirror to ensure you're staying in the right position and maintaining proper technique.

2. Don't swing your back up and down. Once you bend the knees and lean forward at the beginning, hold this position rigidly while your arms do the lifting of the weights.

3. Don't bang the dumbbells together when they come back down and meet at the bottom again. This could easily lead to an injury, so make sure you lower them in a controlled manner as you do in the negative part of most exercises.

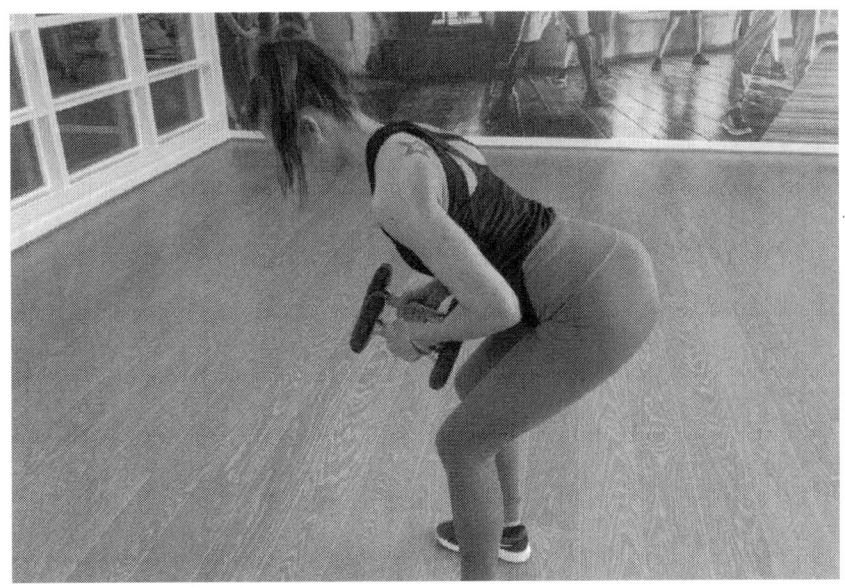

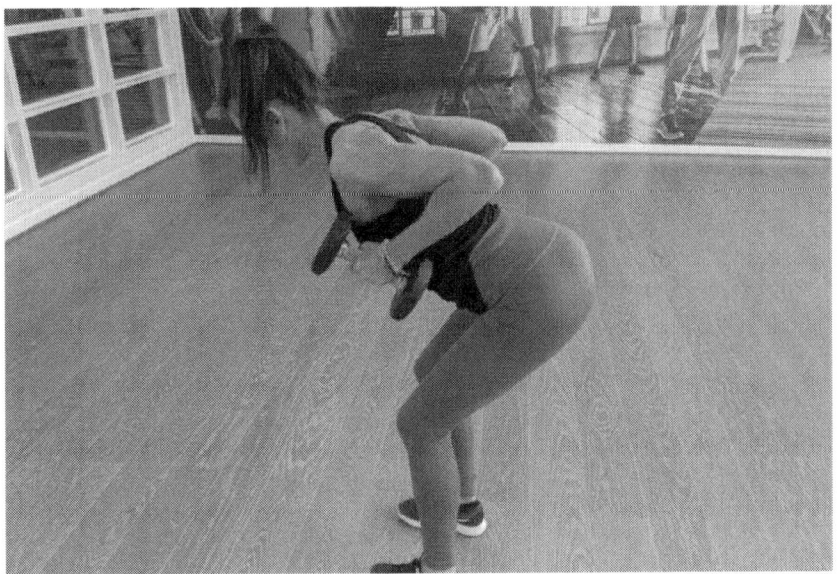

GOBLET SQUATS

Simple squatting exercise while holding a dumbbell.

Muscles worked

Quadriceps, glutes, hamstring, calves.

What to do

1. Stand with your back straight, with your feet slightly wider than hip width, your toes pointing slightly outwards. Hold a kettlebell/dumbbell in both hands close to your chest.

2. Keep your core engaged while looking straight ahead. You want to keep looking ahead, core engaged and back straight throughout the entire movement.

3. Push your hips back and begin bending your knees to perform the squat.

4. Make sure you focus on keeping your chest out and shoulders slightly back as you continue pushing your hips back and squatting down. The main target is to get your hips below parallel with your knees. Taking most of the weight on your heels.

5. Make sure your elbows are tight while holding the dumbbell/kettlebell at the bottom of the movement. Also make sure your knees don't track over your toes.

6. Push up through your heels to return to the starting position. Push your hips forward at the top of the squat to engage your glutes.

What NOT to do

1. Hold the dumbbell/kettlebell to far out from your body – make sure your elbows are bent and the weight is close to your chest.

2. Leaning too far forward or backward – your want the movement to be safe and feel natural and not set you up for injury.

3. Push up onto toes – this can compromise knee integrity and also put you off balance.

4. Allow the knees to track inward – some people have knee valgus and this is a good way to check it. Focus on pushing the legs slightly outwards while performing this move.

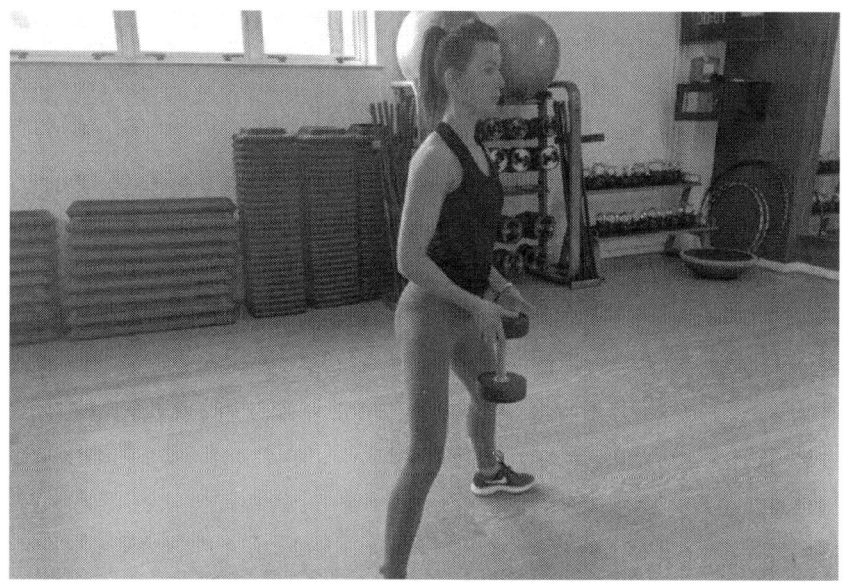

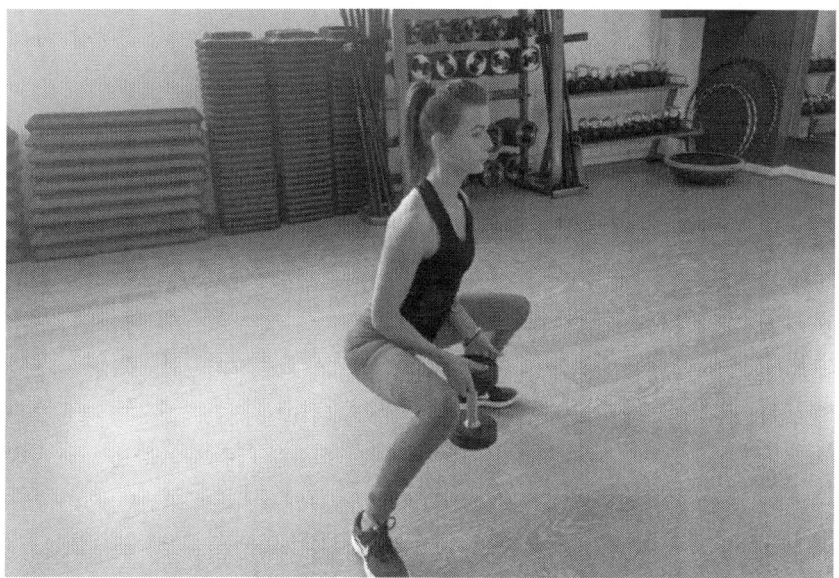

WALKING LUNGES

This is an amazing exercise, which I use most days when training my legs. It helps build strength, stability and endurance. They're also great for developing strong legs.

Muscles worked

Quadriceps, glutes, hamstrings.

What to do

1. Practice this first without weight as getting it right first time can be tricky, aim for good technique and not speed.

2. Keep your back straight, shoulders back and relaxed, core engaged and keep looking forward – pick somewhere in front of you to look at, this distracts you from looking at the floor.

3. Take a step forward with one leg, lowering your hips until both knees are bent at about a 90-degree angle. Ensure your knee is directly above your ankle. Make sure your other knee doesn't touch the floor. Push back up with your heels to the starting position.

4. Continue this movement with alternate legs while walking forward.

5. When you feel ready you can add dumbbells.

6. Hold the dumbbells at each side of your body, try and keep your arms nice and relaxed as this will help the move feel more natural. Repeat as above.

What NOT to do

1. Lean too far forward or backwards, this can put strain on your back.

2. Allow the knee to track over the toes – over time this can damage your joints.

3. Take yourself too seriously – enjoy the process!

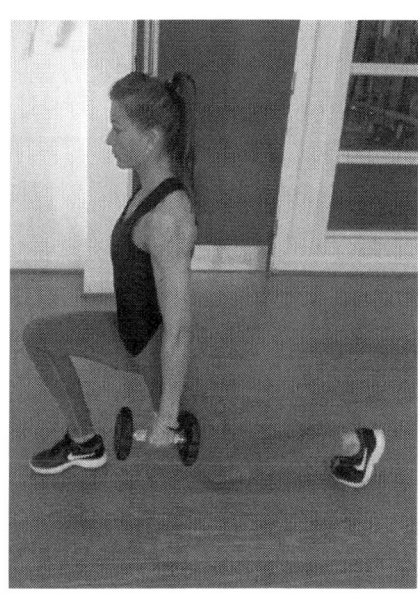 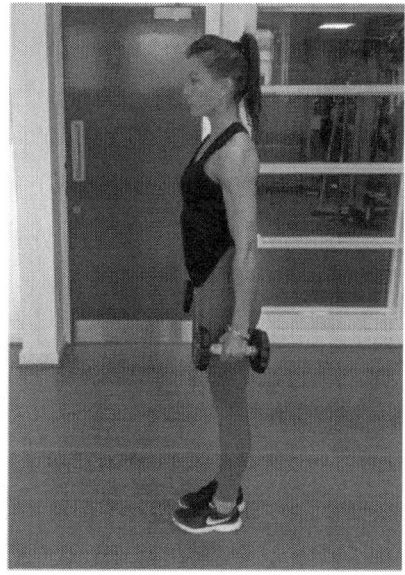

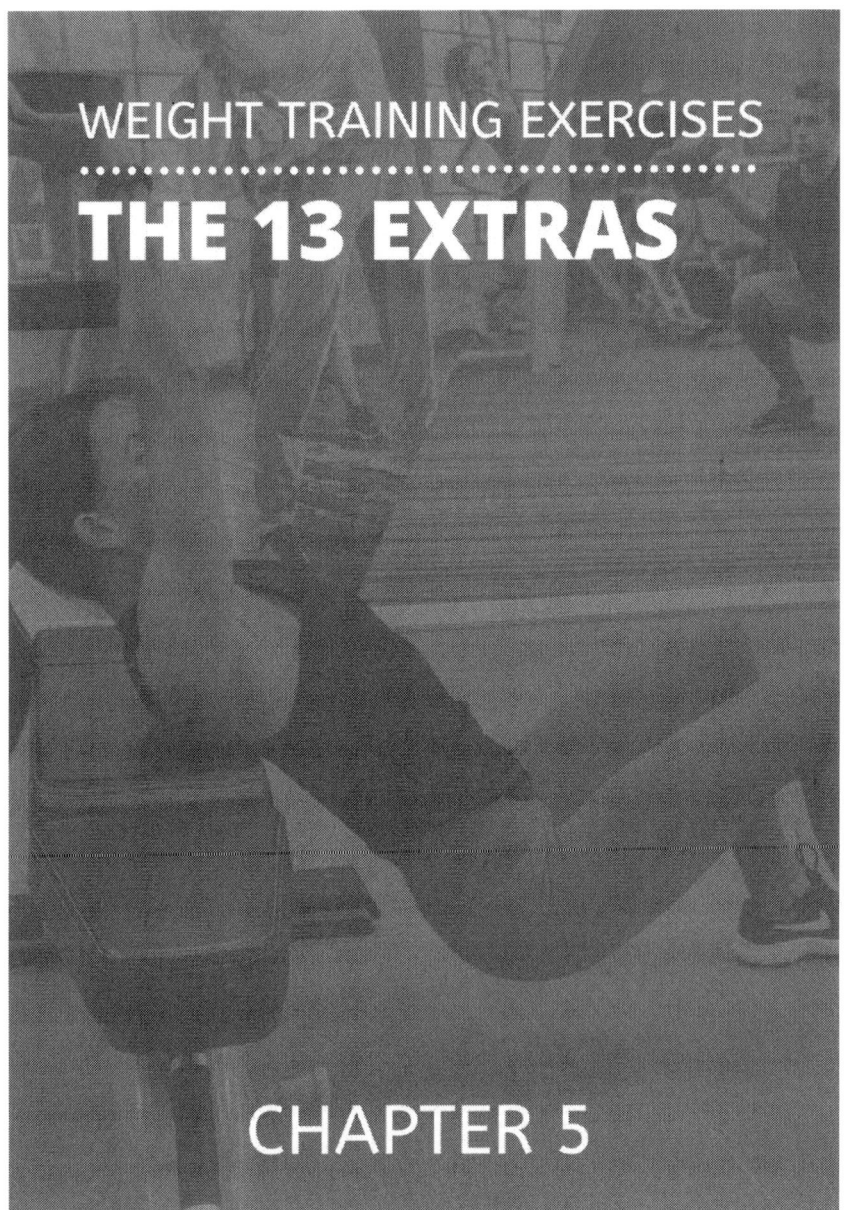

WEIGHT TRAINING EXERCISES

THE 13 EXTRAS

CHAPTER 5

SHOULDER PRESS

This is a straightforward (but not easy) exercise that involves pressing a loaded barbell above your head.

Gym newbies should always begin this exercise using the bar only. As mentioned before the standard weight for an Olympic barbell in gyms is 15kg-20kg, and you shouldn't be adding any weight on until you can do 10-12 with the bar alone.

Muscles worked

Shoulders, arms, trapezius/upper back.

What to do

1. Place the bar on a weights rack at chest height.

2. With your feet planted at hip width underneath the bar, grab the bar with an underhand grip at slightly wider than shoulder width. (This means it should be resting on your palms while your fingers wrap round it tightly).

3. Lift the bar off the rack and on to your upper chest area, before taking a couple of steps back from the rack.

4. With your feet planted in a natural, hip-width position, press the bar directly above your head until your arms lock out at the elbow.

5. Pause for half a second at the top of the move, and then lower the weight back down in a controlled manner until your elbows reach a 90 degree bend.

6. Push the weight back up forcefully until your arms lock out again at the top, and repeat for the duration of the set.

What NOT to do

1. Don't rack the bar too high or too low at the beginning as this will make it difficult to stay balanced as you try to get in the starting position.

2. Don't bend your knees to give yourself an extra push when pressing upwards. The upper half of your body should be doing the work, not the bottom half.

3. Don't look downwards or up at the ceiling when performing this exercise. Stand in front of a mirror and look straight ahead throughout, keeping a close eye on your technique and checking for when your arms reach that 90 degree angle on the way down.

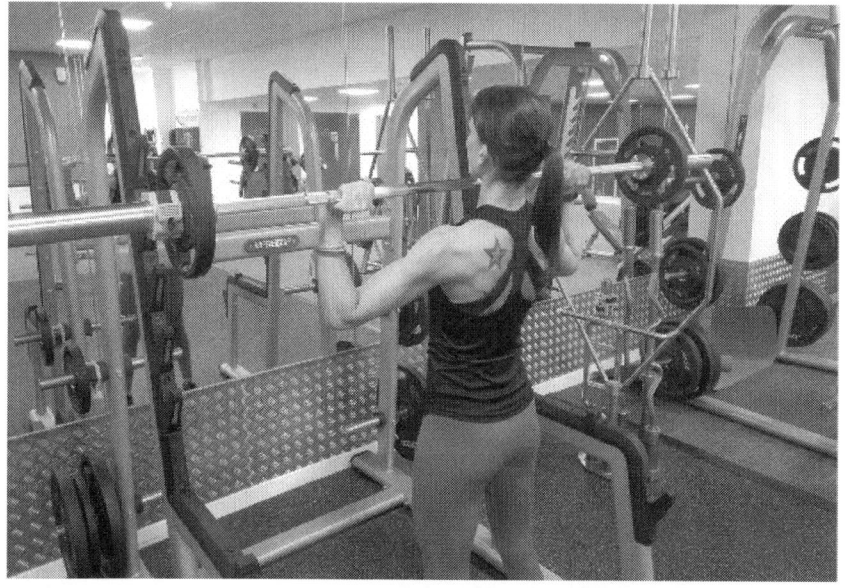

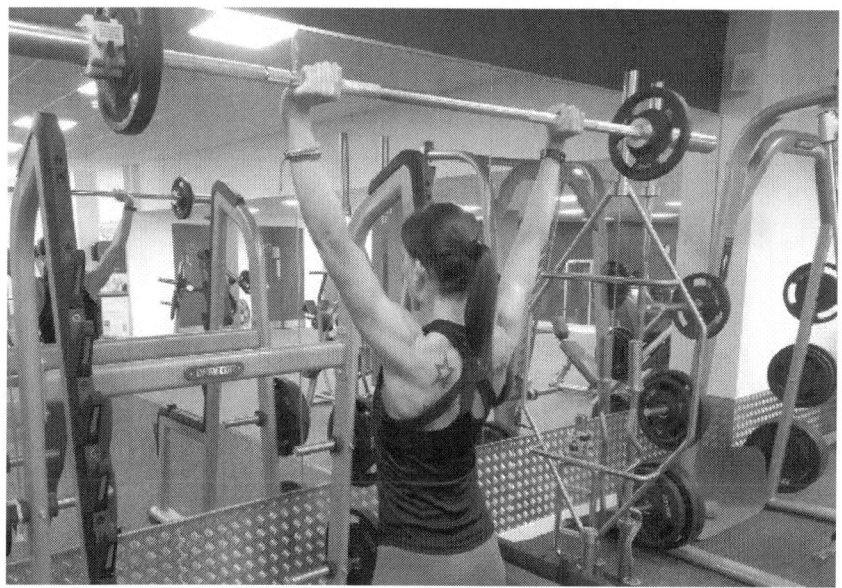

DUMBBELL PULLOVER

An exercise involving a single dumbbell being raised over your head while lying on a bench.

Muscles worked

Chest, shoulders, triceps.

What to do

1. Line a flat bench up next to the dumbbell rack, and then sit down with a dumbbell upright on your lap.

2. Lie back with the dumbbell sitting upright on your chest, and put both palms underneath the top dumbbell plate. Then lock your thumbs round the metal bar in the middle of the dumbbell.

3. Push the dumbbell upwards until your arms are straight, and the dumbbell is raised directly above your upper chest area.

4. Keeping your arms as straight as possible throughout, slowly bring the dumbbell back until your upper arms are in line with your ears.

5. Again keeping your arms as straight and rigid as possible, bring the dumbbell back up to the starting position, squeezing your arms and shoulder muscles for a second as you reach the top. That's one full rep completed.

What NOT to do

1. Don't bend your arms when lowering the dumbbell – keep it a safe distance away from your head.

2. Don't let your arms simply drop backwards, this could cause a shoulder injury. Perform the movement in a controlled manner.

3. Don't stretch too far back with the dumbbell as you'll struggle to raise it again, and increase chances of injury.

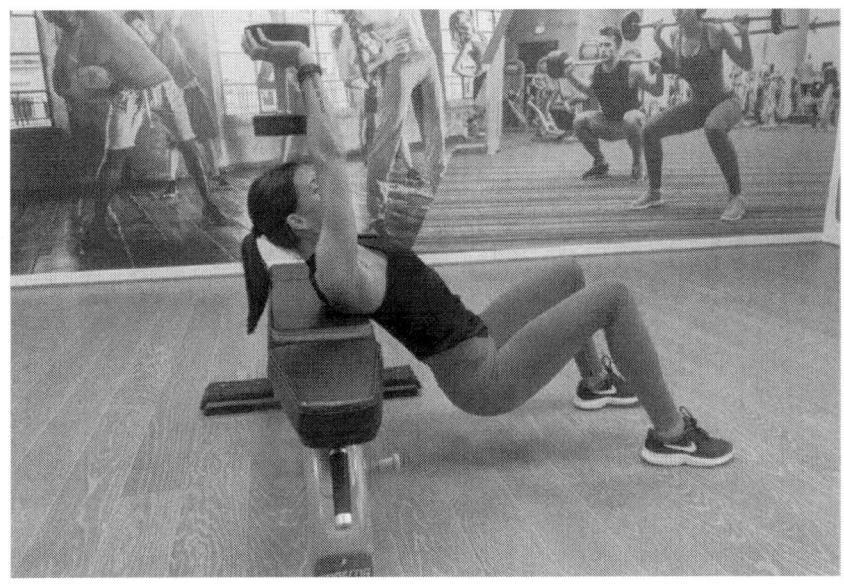

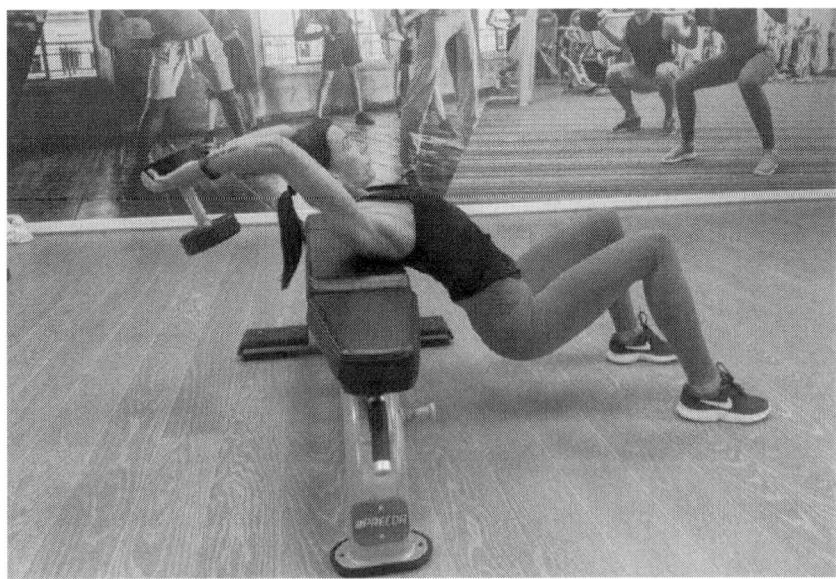

ARNIE PRESS

A dumbbells exercise that targets all muscle in the shoulders.

Muscles worked

Shoulders.

What to do

1. Adjust a weights bench into the upright position.

2. Grab two dumbbells from the rack and sit on the bench, with the dumbbells resting on each knee.

3. Kick each knee upwards, one immediately after the other, to help lift the dumbbells upwards. Then press the dumbbells up in the air until your arms are straight – and your palms are facing outwards.

4. Bring the weights down and outwards, while gradually twisting your arms so that your palms begin to face inwards. (At the halfway point, both palms should be facing each other).

5. As you approach the bottom bring your forearms in to meet each other, and twist the dumbbells in more until you finish with your palms facing completely inwards.

6. Reverse the move, by pushing up and twisting your arms outwards, bit by bit, until they reach the top again with your palms facing outwards again. (See the following pictures).

What NOT to do

1. Don't twist your arms completely at the top, and then lower them. This will result in doing a basic dumbbell shoulder press. You must gradually twist your forearms as you go up and down in this exercise, with your palms finally facing the opposite direction once they reach the top and bottom.

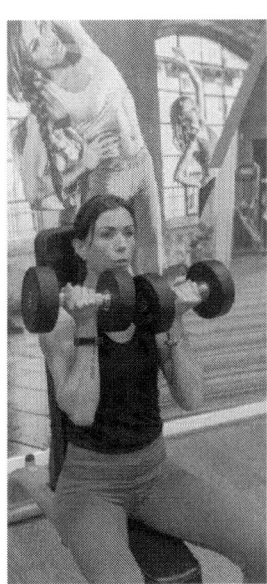 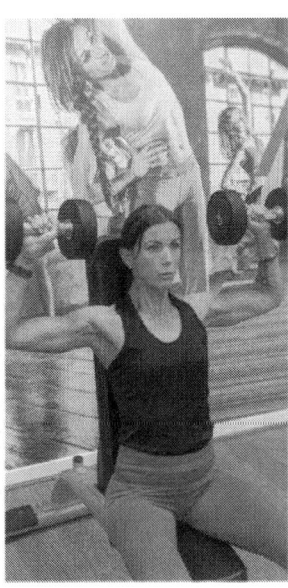 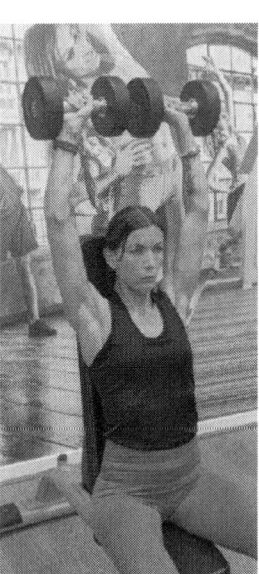

UPRIGHT ROW

A barbell exercise which is best done with an E-z bar (one which has curves in the middle).

Muscles worked

Trapezius, front of shoulders, biceps, forearms.

What to do

1. Place weight discs on either side of an E-z (curved) bar and lock them in place with a safety collar.

2. Grab the bar with a narrow grip, holding each of the two upper grooves like handles.

3. Stand up straight with the bar and keep your feet in the same position, and an upright back posture throughout the exercise.

4. Begin by pulling the bar upwards until it almost reaches your chin. (The E-z bar is better designed for this than a straight bar).

5. Lower the weight back down again until your arms are straight and in the starting position.

What NOT to do

1. Don't use the straight barbell – as this can put unnecessary strain on your wrists.

2. In the second part of the exercise, don't just let the weight flop down immediately. Lower it back down to your thighs area in a controlled way that takes roughly 2 secs.

3. Don't lift the weight only to your lower chest area, lift right up to within a couple of inches of your chin (without smashing it off your chin!)

4. Don't look down at the floor. Get in front of the mirror and keep looking straight ahead, making sure you are bringing the barbell up close enough to your chin.

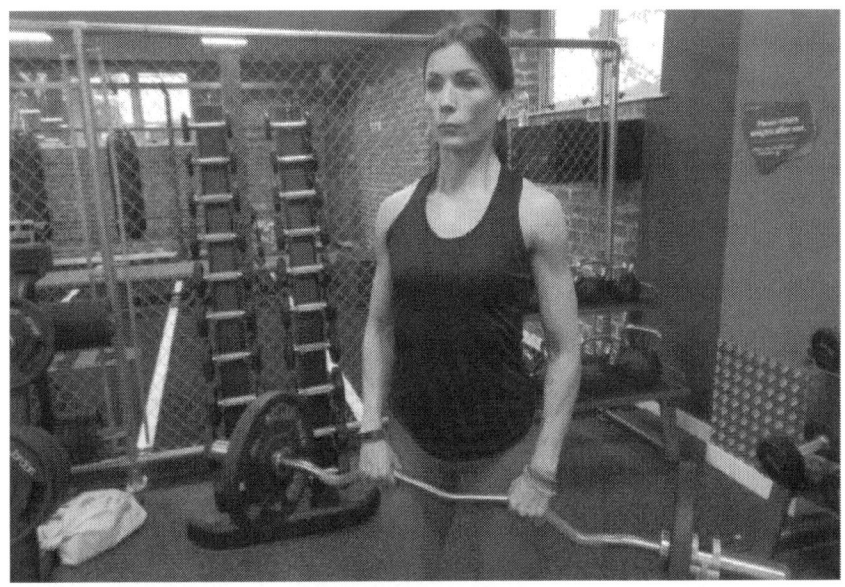

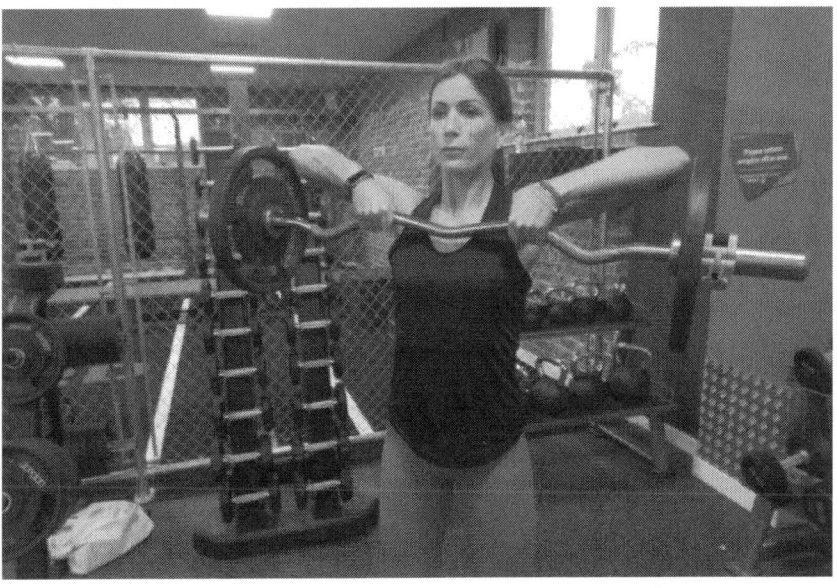

DUMBBELL LATERAL RAISE

A very straightforward, but not easy, dumbbells exercise.

Muscles worked

Shoulders (front and middle), trapezius, core.

What to do

1. Grab a dumbbell in each hand and stand upright with them resting at your sides (palms facing inwards).

2. Keeping your legs and back straight, lift both your arms upwards at the same time until they are straight in a cross position.

3. Lower the dumbbells back down again to your sides in a controlled manner.

What NOT to do

1. Don't swing your body to lift the dumbbells, keep it straight and use your arms to raise the weight.

2. Don't let the dumbbells just drop for the second part of the movement, you definitely don't want them clattering off your hip bones.

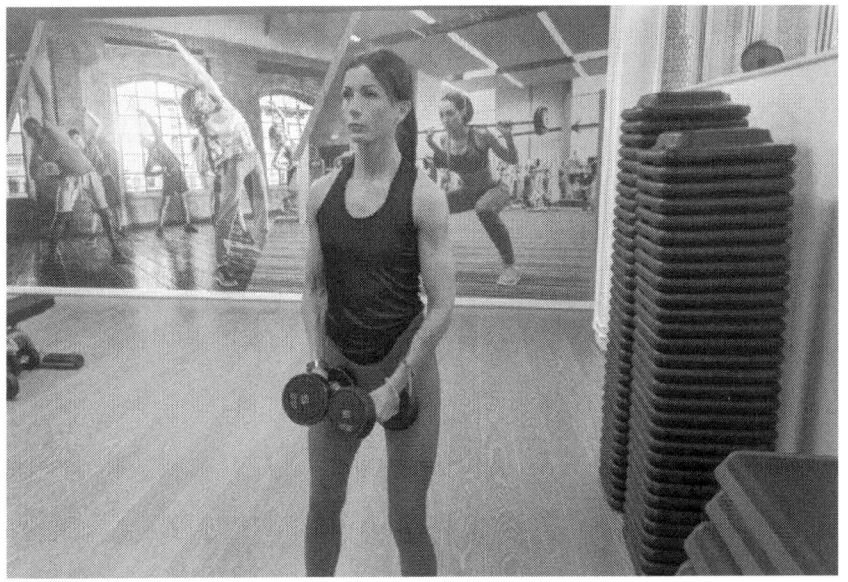

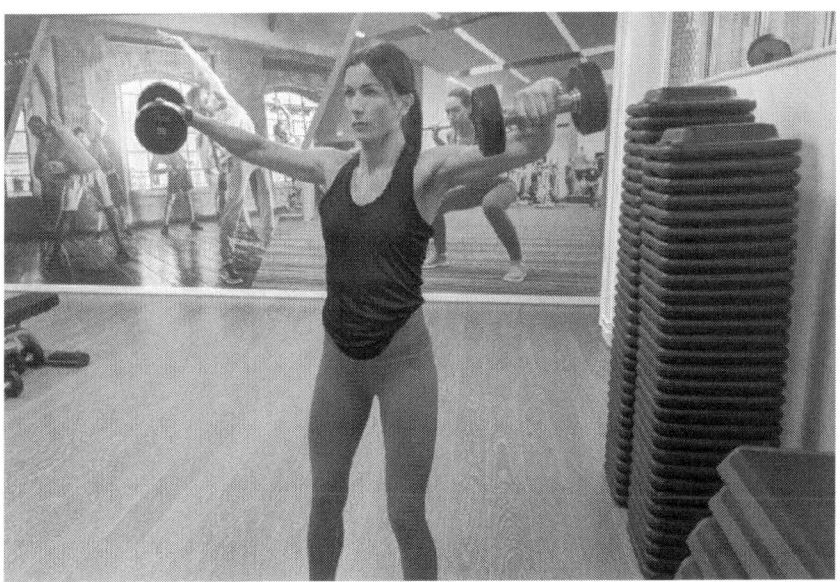

CABLE FLYES

A great exercise involving a cable machine (as you might've guessed) which is great for toning your upper body.

Muscles worked

Shoulders, chest, arms.

What to do

1. Set the pulleys in place at shoulder height at each side of the cable machine. Attach cable handles to each side.

2. Select your chosen level of resistance by putting the pin in place at the machine.

3. Grabbing each cable handle, move forward a couple of steps and lean your upper body forward slightly in order to tauten the cables.

4. At this starting point, your feet should be planted at shoulder width and your arms stretched backwards behind you with the cable handles.

5. With your palms facing in the way, pull the cables inwards in a circular motion until they meet in the middle around a metre from your chest.

6. Bring the cable handles back to the starting position in a controlled manner.

What NOT to do

1. Don't allow your arms to just flop backwards after they meet in the middle. Keep the tension on the cables and release them backwards carefully.

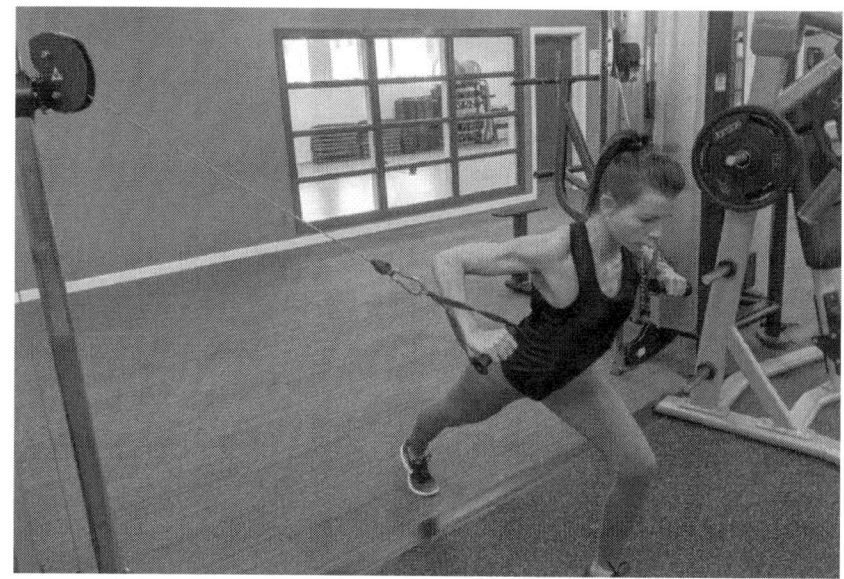

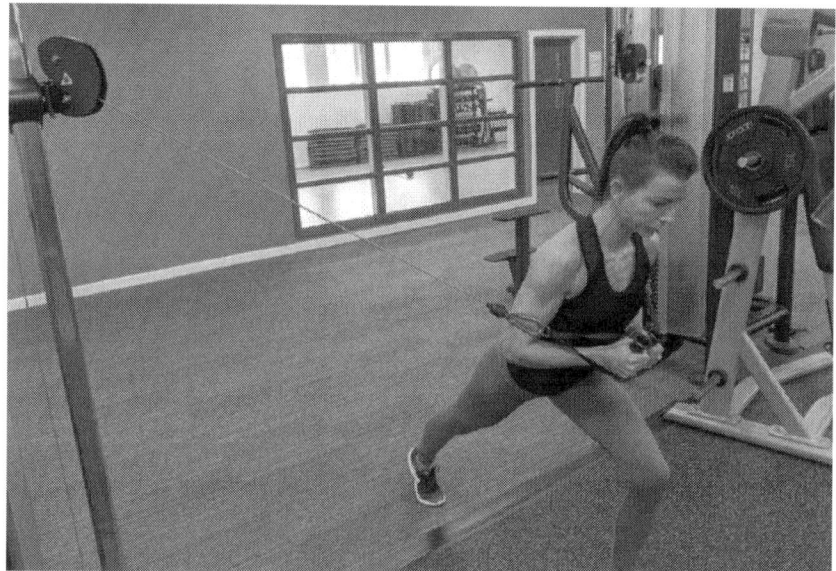

DISC RAISE

A straightforward exercise involving a round weight disc/plate, your hands and shoulders.

Muscles worked

Front of shoulders, chest.

What to do

1. Stand upright with your feet slightly wider than shoulder width apart, and grab hold of a circular weights disc in the middle at either side.

2. Get into position by holding the disc directly in front of your with your arms straight.

3. Keeping your arms straight, raise the disc upwards until it reaches the top of your head.

4. Then bring the disc back down again to shoulder height, always keeping your arms straight throughout.

What NOT to do

1. Don't swing your body to gain any momentum, always keep your feet planted in the one position and your back upright.

2. Don't simply drop the weight back down after you reach the top; it should be a controlled lowering that takes 1-2 secs.

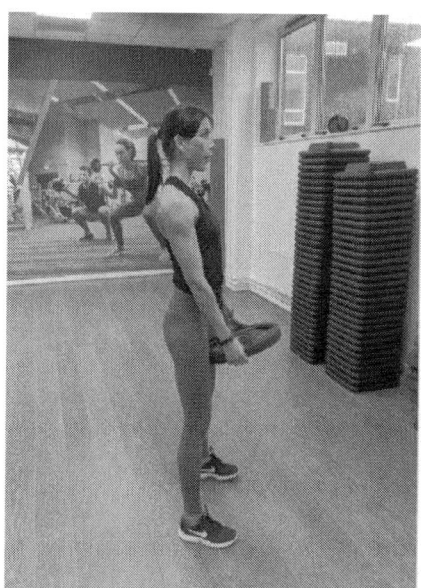 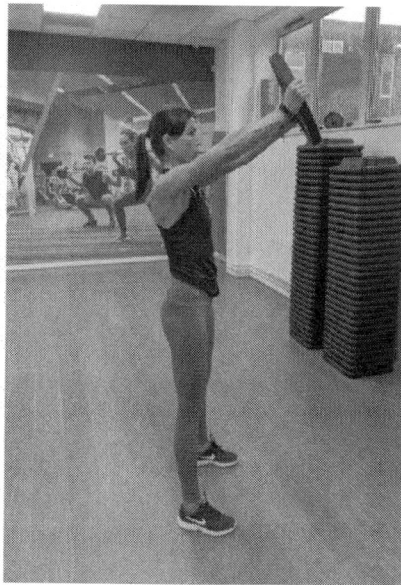

PRESS-UPS

I know, I know...press-ups are hard as hell at the beginning. Not everyone can do proper repetitions at the beginning. That's why I'm going to describe a beginner version, and then a more advance way of doing press-ups.

Muscles worked

Front of shoulders, chest, triceps, core, glutes.

What to do - beginners

1. Kneel down on a floor mat, with your back straight and hands on the floor at slightly wider than shoulder width.

2. Looking directly at the floor below you, bend your arms until they reach a 90 degree angle – or as close to this as you can manage.

3. Press back upwards until your arms are straight and lock out at the elbow.

4. Repeat for as many repetitions as possible, and always try to do at least one more rep than before each time you do these press-ups. Once you can manage 12-15 using your knees for assistance, it's time to try proper press-ups with your legs straight.

What to do – more advanced

1. Find yourself a mat on the gym floor and get into the press-up position, with your feet apart at one end and hands slightly wider than shoulder width at the top end.

2. Keep your body as flat and rigid as possible before beginning the exercise (i.e. don't have your bum high in the air), and keep looking directly at the floor below you.

3. Bend your arms until they reach a 90 degree angle, and then push back upwards forcefully until your arms lock out at the elbow.

4. Repeat for as many repetitions as possible. Tip – do 3 x sets, with 1 minute rest in between, and count the total number of repetitions at the end. Each time you do press-ups try to beat your score record by at least 1 more press-up.

What NOT to do

1. Don't lower your hips down only and not bend the arms. The emphasis should be on the arms doing the work and lowering the rest of your body downwards.

2. Don't do half reps by bending the arms just slightly. Five reps with good technique is better than 15 with poor form.

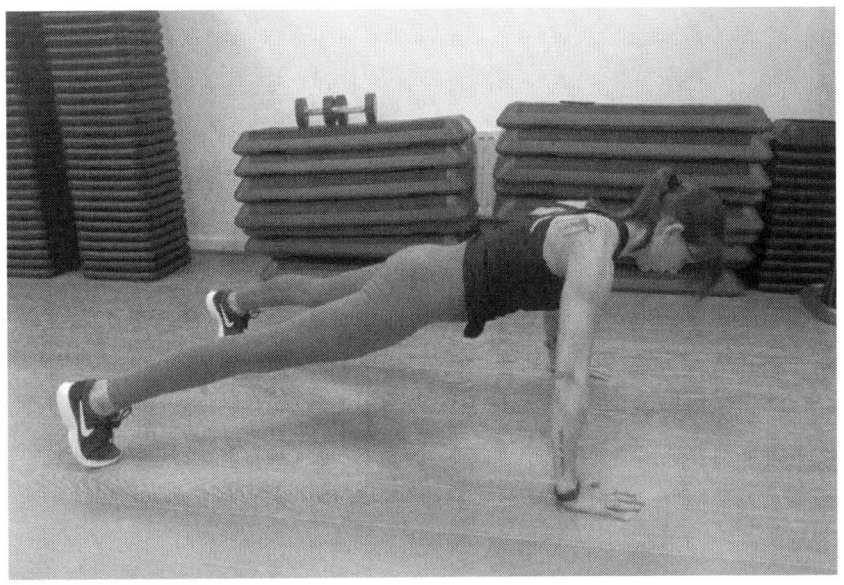

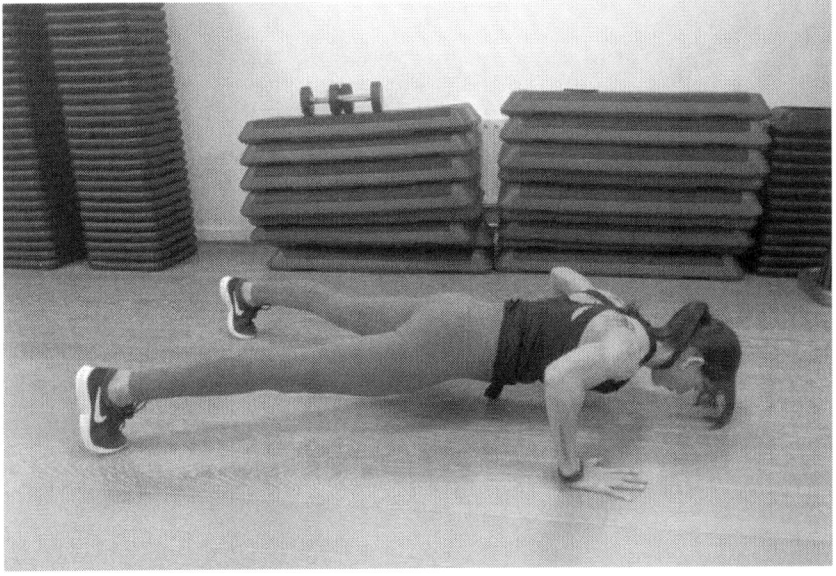

HAMSTRING CURLS

A machine exercise like no other for tightening the back of your legs. The hamstring machine has weights attached to a cable and you take a seat to do the lifting.

Muscles worked

Hamstrings.

What to do

1. First adjust the lever at the front of the machine so that it's raised up in the air.

2. Put the pin in the machine at a weights level that's suitable for you. You might to experiment to find the sweet spot.

3. Sit down on the machine, with your back resting against the seat behind. Slide your lower legs in between the two cushions until your legs are in a straight position outwards.

Your heels (not your calves) should be resting on top of the lower cushion and your shins pushing against the upper cushion.

** You may have to adjust the lever and seat behind you to get into the right position as described above.

4. There are usually handles at either side of the machine's seat. Grab onto these with your hands and continue to keep your back firmly pushed against the seat back support behind you.

5. Using your heels, kick the lower cushion downwards until the soles of your feet are parallel with the floor.

6. Feel the squeeze on your hamstring for just a moment, before releasing the weighted cushion back to the top in a controlled manner.

What NOT to do

1. Don't begin the exercise until your legs and back are in the proper position; as described in point three above.

2. Don't simply let go of the squeeze at the bottom of the exercise as the machine will throw your legs upwards, and could possibly cause an injury. Your legs should also be working in this second part of the movement with a controlled release of the weights back to the top.

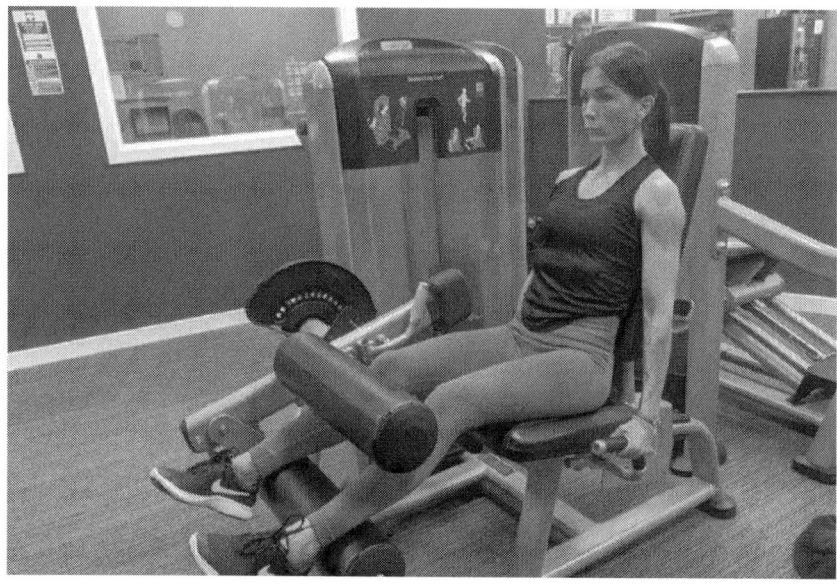

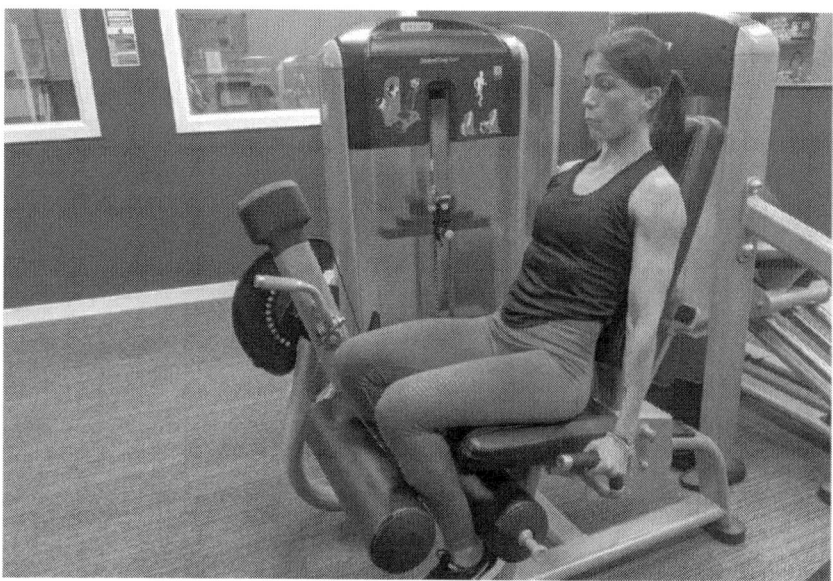

BACK EXTENSION

This exercise gets the blood pumping to your glutes and assists with strength for the bigger exercises such as squats, deadlifts and hip thrusts.

Muscles worked

Glutes, hamstrings.

What to do

1. Lay across the machine with head and neck in a neutral position. Position your feet at a 45 degree angle, as seen in the pictures.

2. Tuck your chin in and slightly round your upper back – this helps to lengthen the hamstrings and glutes.

3. Lean forward – you don't need a huge amount of extension here, just enough to feel a stretch.

4. Pause for a second and engage the glutes (squeeze your butt cheeks).

5. Keep them engaged while driving back to starting position.

6. Keep upper back slightly rounded as this will activate the glutes and put less pressure on the lower back.

What NOT to do

1. Over arch your back – keep that upper back slightly rounded at all times

2. Over stretch on the decend – again this can be dangerous for your lower back depending on flexibility.

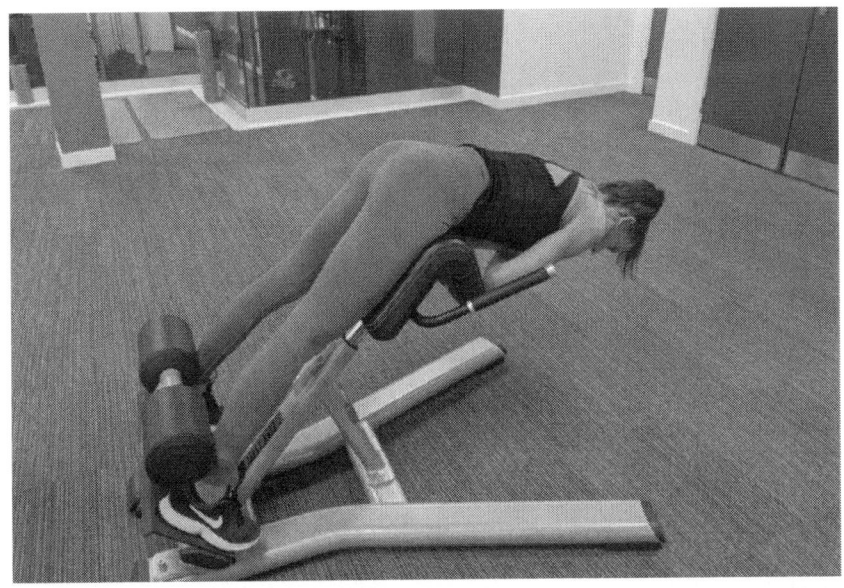

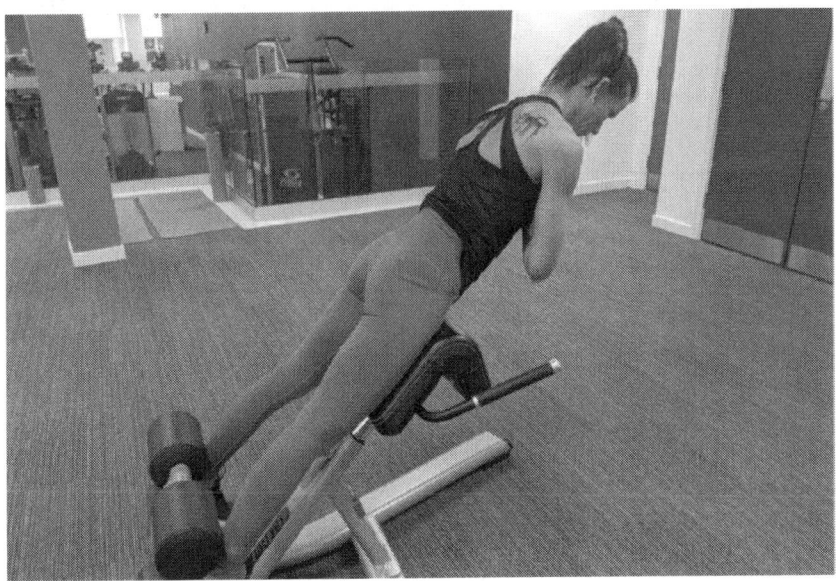

GLUTE HAM KICKBACK

Glute ham kickbacks with loop bands are incredibly effective at isolating your glutes and hamstrings. You'll need a resistance band for this one.

Muscles worked

Glutes, hamstrings, quadriceps.

What to do

1. Place a loop band around your thighs.

2. Start in an all fours position and tighten your core.

3. Lift one leg up to a full hip extension and squeeze your glutes at the top.

4. Slowly lower your leg back down to the starting kneeling position. Repeat and then switch legs.

* Contract your glutes hard and keep them clenched at the top of the movement for a prolonged period to maximise results.

What NOT to do

1. Arch your back – make sure you keep core tight.

2. Lean to either side, keep as central as you possibly can.

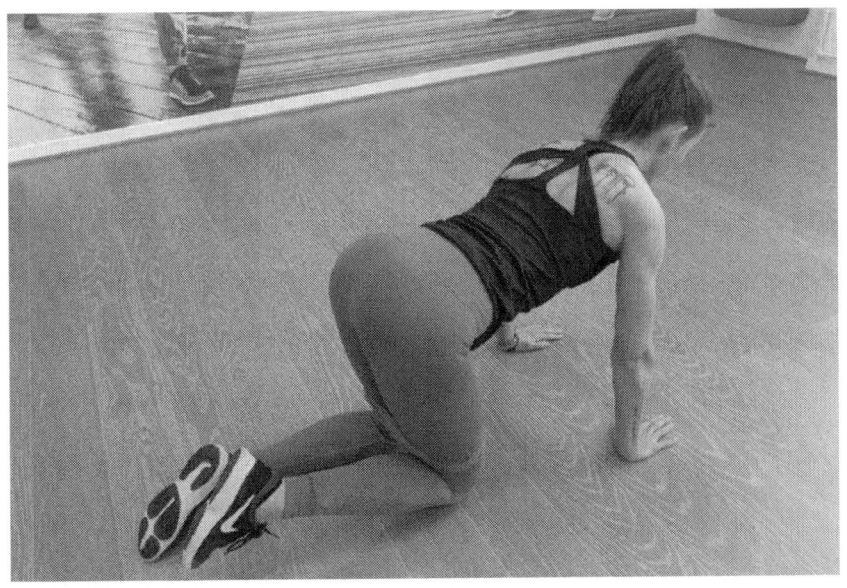

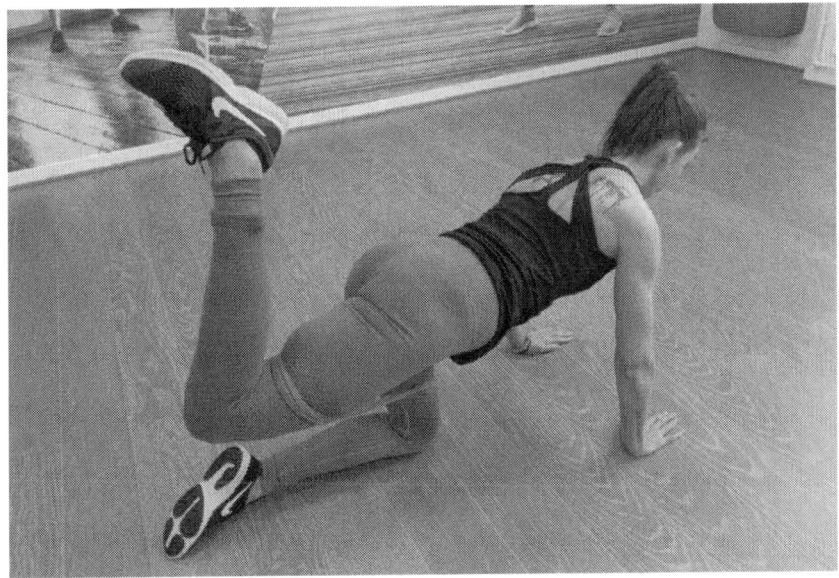

CURTSY SQUATS

We've all done a curtsy at one point in our lives, and now it's time to do a fair few of them in the gym to develop strong legs.

While it's so effective for toned legs, it's also quite difficult to master at first. I suggest practicing the move without a weight at first, and then add a barbell in once you're ready.

Muscles worked

Glutes, hamstrings, core, quadriceps, calves.

What to do

1. Pick up a barbell with both hands and lift over your head and rest it on your shoulder blades (just like in a starting position for squats).

2. As you lower your body, pick one foot off the floor and cross it behind your other leg.

3. As you slowly lower your body, tap the behind leg on the floor before rising up again and placing your feet in the starting position.

What NOT to do

1. Go too heavy with the weight, or even add weight until you're comfortable with the technique.

2. Do the exercise too close to other people. You need enough space to move from side to side, and don't want to bang into other people when performing the exercise.

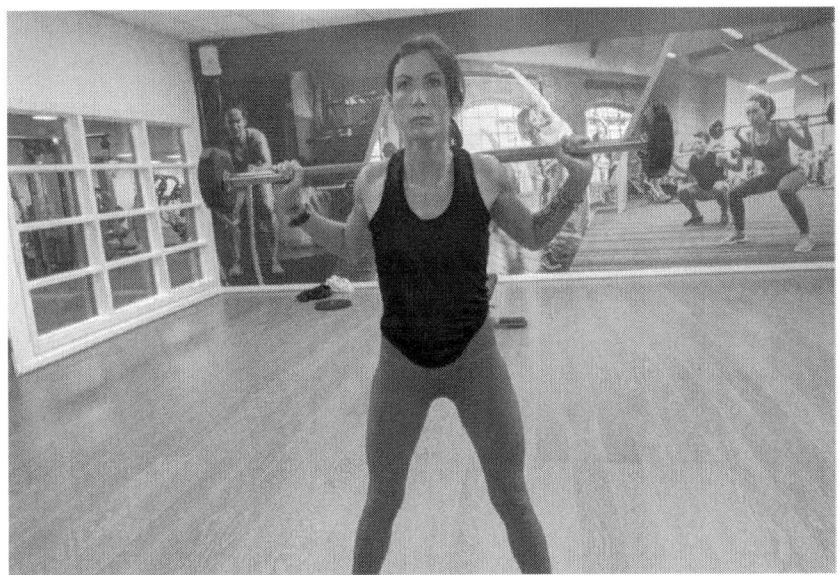

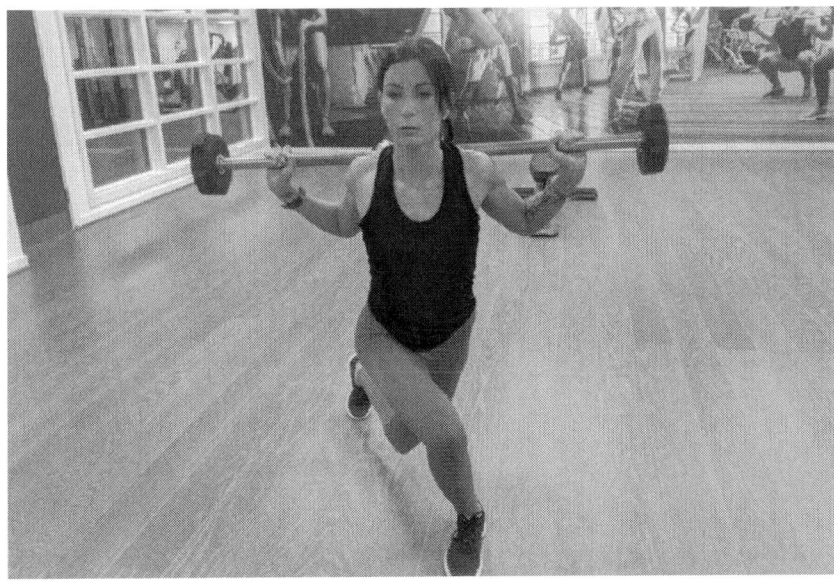

SPLIT SQUATS

Relax...you don't really have to do the splits. This is another excellent exercise for adding some serious definition to your legs. Once you're comfortable and more experienced with these, you can do the exercise while holding dumbbells in each hand.

Muscles worked

Quadriceps, glutes, hamstrings.

What to do

1. Start by standing about two feet in front of a bench or step.

2. Lift one leg up behind you and place the top of your foot on the bench or step. Your feet should still be shoulder-width apart and the other foot should be far enough in front of the bench so that you can comfortably lunge.

3. Tighten your core, lean slightly forward at the waist, beginning to lower down and bending the knee into a lunge position.

4. Push up through your standing foot, using the power from your quads and hamstrings to return to standing.

What NOT to do

1. Lean back, slightly forward is key - and engaging your core.

2. Push your knees outwards or inwards. Keep them centred throughout.

3. Drive your knee forward over your toes as this will set you up for injury.   If your knee goes over your toes the start again and readjust.

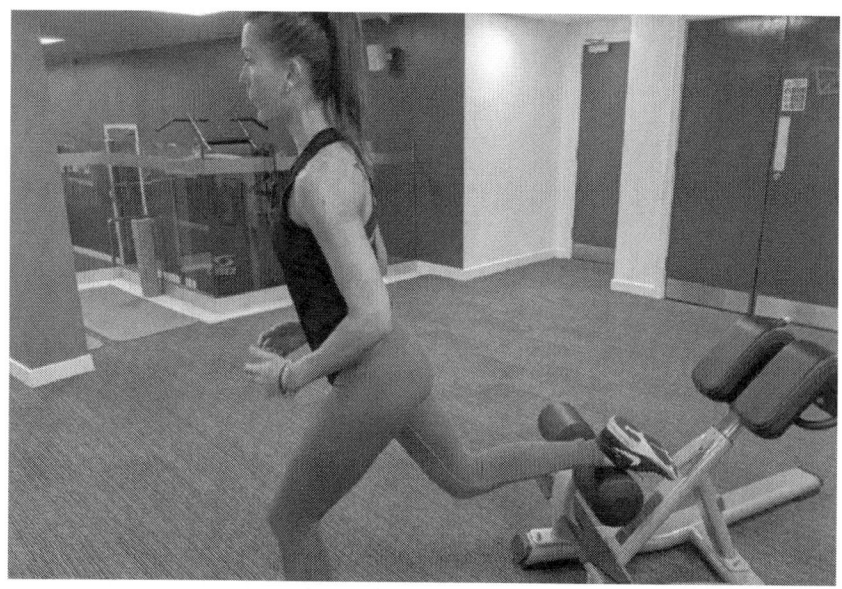

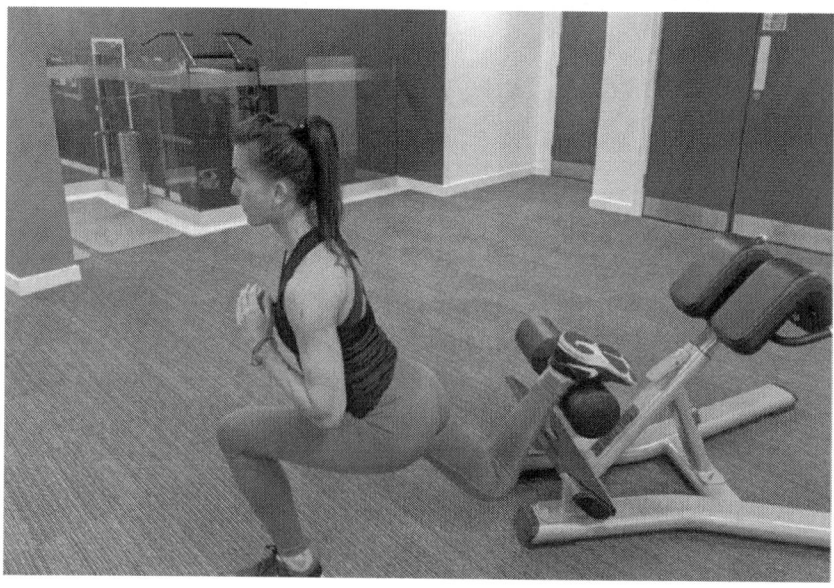

Chapter 6

Creating A Workout Plan

We all do this one thing every day girls, without really thinking about it.

Putting make-up on in the morning. Fixing your hair before before work. Picking the right outfit and shoes for a night out. Getting in the food shopping.

We always prepare, prepare, prepare. So why not do the same when it comes to your workouts?

Our life is organised in every other department to make everything go smoothly, yet most of us are half-hearted about fitness. If you don't have a clear plan of attack for your gym workouts, then you're going to be unfocused and won't push yourself hard enough.

From previous chapters, we already know the types of exercises you should be doing. But how many exercises should you do per workout? How long should your workouts be? What about rest periods? Is there a danger of over-training?

These are questions you might have, and we'll deal with them all as we cover exactly how to prepare properly for the gym by creating your workout plans.

No more turning up at the gym hoping that it's not busy and just hopping on whatever machine is free. That kind of approach will get you nowhere.

"By failing to prepare, you are preparing to fail," – you've likely heard this phrase before, and it's absolutely true.

Now it's time to get serious about getting you in great shape, and an important part of that is mapping out your workouts before you even walk through those gym doors.

Preparing For Your Weights Workouts

Let's quickly outline an ideal weight training workout plan for you, then we'll going into the specifics of getting down to work in the gym.

Workouts per week: Ideally, go to the gym 4 days per week. Any more than that can hinder progress as your body needs sufficient rest in order to change, tone and develop lean muscle.

I previously made the mistake of weightlifting every day and becoming so fatigued that it resulted in injury.

Yeah it feels good pushing yourself, and I do believe that everyone has it in them to do some form of exercise on a daily basis, but be aware that this can be detrimental to your health and wellbeing overall.

Getting in four weights workouts over the course of a week, with recovery periods in between, will move you nicely towards your goals.

Workout duration – you don't have to do long, gruelling workouts to get best results. In terms of time spent in the gym, I try and be in and out in around an hour.

Something that can really keep your workouts efficient is doing what's known as 'supersets', which basically involves doing two exercises in pairs in quick succession. It essentially means you squeeze in a maximum amount of exercises in the shortest amount of time. We'll go into more detail about supersets later.

But when you first start lifting weights don't be too concerned with time, it's not actually an indicator of how well you've trained. Some people can spend two hours in the gym and get little out of it (usually because they're not lifting weights like us).

Variety – you'll be glad to know that your workouts should always be changing. Let's be honest, we've all got bored of following the same old routine before.

When I first started lifting weights, I completed the same workout over and over...until my brain almost exploded with boredom.

Here's what to do instead: choose different exercises each time you train in the gym, mix up the order of those exercises, and always try to throw your body a curveball every now and again to keep challenging yourself.

Exercise selection – firstly, I'd recommend doing 9-11 exercises in your workouts. In the previous chapters we covered my 13 Fundamentals and 13 Extras – a total of 26 brilliant exercises you can choose from.

It's simply a case of you picking exercises from each of these two categories, and mixing and matching. By doing so, you'll ensure there's always variety, as mentioned above, and your body won't get used to the same old routine.

By taking on fresh, challenging workouts you'll make even more progress towards your goals of lean muscle and fat loss.

Keeping on track – I highly recommend writing down all the exercise you're going to do in advance. Jot them down in a small diary, or use a notes app on your mobile phone like I do.

If I'm going to train early morning, then I make sure I complete the exercise list the night before. This means you're organised and motivated to get going in the gym the next day.

Each workout plan, written down in black and white, will also help keep you on track. You won't forget exercises in the gym, and you should also write down how much weight you've been lifting alongside each exercise, along with the number of reps you manage.

Getting Down To Work In The Gym

Everything I've just described will give you a firm foundation for fitness success, but of course no results can come until you take action in the gym.

We'll now go over five key elements of your weight training workouts, and how to get the numbers right in order to fatigue your muscles effectively and increase fat burning.

#1 Exercises

As already mentioned, you'll have chosen 9-11 exercises for each workout.

#2 Repetitions

Aim for between 9 and 12 repetitions of each of those exercises. If you can hit 13 reps then you need to increase the weight, whereas if you're only managing less than 8 reps, then the weight needs to be reduced.

The important thing is how much you push yourself to complete that last rep.

#3 Sets of each exercise

Between 3 and 4 sets of each exercise is sufficient to work the muscles hard, triggering development and raising your metabolism levels too for more fat loss.

#4 Rest period

When it come to taking a break in between each set of an exercise, I recommend keeping it short. There's loads of research out there to say that woman recover quicker from physical exercise than men.

Sorry to offend the guys, but it's true. It's all to do with our genetic make-up.

When resting between exercise sets, it's best to wait no longer than a minute. This keeps the heart rate slightly elevated and optimises fat burning.

#5 Training methods

You can apply all of the above – exercises, repetitions, sets, and rest period – into two straightforward training methods.

One – you can do each of your exercises one after the other, set by set, with the recommended 1 minute rest period in between.

Two – you can do those 'super-sets' we touched upon earlier. Super-sets involve pairing two exercises together and doing them in quick succession with only 20-30 secs rest in between each one.

For example, your workout could look like this:

Super-set 1: Squats, 20-30 secs rest, then do military press. Have 1 minute rest, then repeat. Do this 3-4 times in total.

Super-set 2: Upright row, 20-30 secs rest, then do bent over row. Have 1 minute rest, then repeat. Again do this 3-4 times in total.

Super-sets 3, 4 & 5: Barbell curls/reverse flyes; Bench press/cable row; curtsy squats/dumbbell lunges, all following the same process as above.

Warning: super-sets are not easy, but they're guaranteed to work your muscles hard and the lack of rest helps increase fat burning further. They're essentially a hybrid version of weight training and HIIT.

It can be mentally and physically exhausting during the workouts at times, but it is well worth it for the confidence and sense of achievement you gain afterwards.

Incase It Doesn't All Go To Plan...Have A Back-Up Plan

Always, always, always...I can't stress this enough...have a backup plan. Let me explain why.

Say you've prepared your workout plan, got your gym gear ready, selected your favourite training music playlist, arrived at the gym...and you discover the place is mobbed!

This is a common problem and it could easily derail your workout plan for the day. When you can't use any of the equipment that you had planned for exercises 1, 2, or 3, because they're already being used, you can feel deflated.

Don't drop your head down – and don't quit! You can always find a way to work around it. Warm up well while equipment is being used, change the order of the exercises you have planned, perhaps ask someone if you can jump in during their rest period.

Seeing the gym really busy makes it easy to make up excuses and only do a half-hearted workout, or simply to turn around and walk out the door again.

Just don't stress, it all works out in the end, trust me. If you're determined, then you'll make the situation work for you.

Below are a few key gym essentials to remember, which will also help ensure your workout plans go ahead without any issues:

* Your list of exercises in a pocket diary or saved on your mobile phone.

* A mobile phone that is actually charged.

* Earphones for your favourite gym tunes.

* A decent playlist, one that gets you fired up. For me, in the gym it's got to be some AC/DC, RnB or techno.

* A water bottle.

13 Workout Mistakes Not To Make

We all make mistakes on our health and fitness journey, I've certainly made plenty along the way. I've flagged up some of the most common ones – so that you don't have to make them too.

1. Doing the same boring routine over and over – remember to keep changing things up for each workout, swapping exercises in and out.

2. Forgetting your earphones – sounds trivial, but no music will drop your motivation levels and might well ruin your workout.

3. Forgetting your gym gear – there's nothing more annoying than turning up at the gym after work, raring to go, and then realising you forgot your clothes. Check and double check before leaving the house.

4. Lifting too light – this means there won't be enough strain on your muscles to grow strength and develop lean muscle.

5. Lifting too heavy – remember that if you can't manage 8 repetitions, then decrease the weight.

6. Falling over – easily done if you don't concentrate on your exercise technique properly.

7. Dropping a plate on someone's foot – also easily done if you don't use safety collars on barbells and plates slide off.

8. Getting 'pinned' under a bar – be careful with the bench press as this happened to me. Go light at first, and get someone to watch over you as you progressively lift heavier.

9. Wasting too much time on cardio – put your focus on weight training as it not only burns fat like cardio, but has the added bonus of toning your muscles at the same time.

10. Spending 2-3 hours in the gym – there's no need if you following the training advice I described earlier in this chapter.

11. Spending 15 minutes in the gym – that's when you know you're pretending at this health and fitness game.

12. Overtraining – stick to the 4 training days per week, and get sufficient rest, to avoid over-exertion.

13. Going in with no workout plan – the main thrust of this entire chapter. If you plan to get great fitness results, then you've got to plan ahead.

Chapter 7

How To Stay Committed To Your Goals

The biggest block to your fitness success is not quite what you think it is.

Too many women get caught up in extreme diets, new workout programmes that excite them for a week or two, or counting every calorie.

But there are three factors which often throw a spanner in the works, and limit progress:

#1 Unrealistic goals (i.e. thinking you can achieve a super toned, model body in 6 weeks, if you just train hard every day).

#2 Putting too much pressure on yourself (to the point where you can become stressed about a fitness programme you should actually be enjoying).

#3 Being impatient (transforming your body shape takes time and serious effort, you've got to have patience).

I have three words for you that will counter those three problems above: <u>enjoy the journey</u>.

My dad died when I was 20, but I still clearly remember what he used to say to me when I was younger whenever I became impatient.

"Victoria, if you want to build a wall, you don't simply put up an entire wall and that's it," he told me. "You gather everything you need, and build that wall one brick at time. The hard work and effort you put in will feel even more rewarding in the end."

When I feel disheartened I always remember his voice saying those words to me and I remind myself that change can take time. Like most people, we want everything done instantly.

Just please remember that this is a process for you to enjoy, one step at a time. Think in terms of a long game, but you still get to make progress each step of the way – steadily becoming a stronger and better you.

A New Lifestyle, Not A New Programme

How long should you commit to a weight training programme for? How soon can you expect to see results? How can you stay on track if your motivation usually dwindles? (Like it does for most of us).

Firstly, if you create workouts and lift weights the way I described earlier, then training like this in the gym can become a healthy lifestyle change that can be ongoing, rather than simply doing a programme for a set amount of time and then walking away.

My hope with this book is to convince people like you that weight training can be transformational for you physically, mentally and bring you a new level of confidence you probably never have had before.

When that happens, you become hooked on weight training – and 3-4 gym sessions becomes a natural part of your weekly routine. It's not like dragging yourself to fitness classes you don't particularly enjoy, you'll actually be excited for every weight training session.

This is exactly what I've experienced, as have several of my friends. I want the same for you.

In terms of how long it takes to see results, it all depends on exactly what you're looking to achieve. But of course, it's not the same for everyone as our bodies are all different and there are various factors, such as age and gym experience, that will influence your progress.

It could take a 22-year-old woman who is fairly active 7-8 weeks to see clear results in terms of changing her body shape, i.e. more toned arms and legs, and improving the shape of her bum.

Meanwhile, it could take a 57-year-old heavily overweight woman a bit longer because she is new to the gym, and has a lot of excess bodyfat to lose first before toning up her body overall.

But the bottom line is: weight training does work – if you put in the work.

But that doesn't mean it's a case of you 'have to do this'. It's more like you 'get to do this'.

Exercising this way, you can achieve more muscle tone and fat loss at the same time.

Exercising this way, you can increase your strength levels exponentially.

By exercising this way, you'll actually make your body more efficient at burning fat. This is because for every pound of muscle you develop, your body automatically burns 35-50 more calories just to maintain it.

And while I'm advising you that your overall fitness goals may take a little longer than you expect to help you stay patient and committed, you absolutely can see positive changes every single week.

I'm talking about:

- Feeling stronger week by week
- Setting new records for numbers of repetitions of exercises and weights levels
- Increased confidence
- Burst of enthusiasm in and outside of the gym
- People commenting on the changes in you

Focus On Organisation, Not Motivation

Motivation levels are always high when we get started on a new fitness or nutrition plan. But let's be honest, those levels can drop pretty quickly when life gets in the way.

You know what I mean. Working later than you expected and feeling drained, having to do the school run, meeting up with friends, taking kids to their sports clubs, and 2,093 other tasks that pile up for us women on a weekly basis.

So yeah, I'm not going to bullshit you and pretend that simply working on staying motivated will keep you on track. Instead of focusing on motivation, pay attention to organisation.

- **Schedule your workouts in advance** – set out the days and specific times you plan on working out. I know it can be hard sometimes if you're a busy mum, but you've got to find time as your workouts are an important part of your self-care, physically and mentally.
- **Adjust your workout plans if need be** – can't make it to the gym four days per week? Then go for three days instead. Not got a full hour to spare for Wednesday's training session? Then do super-sets like I described earlier. You could cut your workout time by 15-20 mins doing this.
- **Go through the motions if necessary** – some days you simply won't be feeling in the mood for the gym, but that's exactly the reason for turning up. Throw your gym gear in a bag, jump in the car and, even if you're still not feeling it

when you arrive at the gym, just go through the motions. You'll be surprised how working your muscles with weights changes your mood and you'll feel a heightened sense of satisfaction after the gym because you pushed through even when you didn't feel like it.

- **Always follow your workout plan** – as described earlier, the workout plan you created will help keep you on track. If your motivation levels are lower and you go into the gym without a plan, it's likely you'll only do half of what you really should be doing. Then you might beat yourself up about it afterwards. Whereas your training plan will keep you organised and focused, no matter how motivated you are.

Also, it's important to remember why you started. Remember you're not a quitter and you want to see this through. And remember all the things you've already accomplished in life, goals that seemed difficult at first, but you still got there.

It's time to apply that courage and strength you have to taking on this new weight training challenge. The fact that you're even reading this book is a first action step towards positively changing your life.

You may only be reading words on these pages, but you're equipping yourself with some important fitness knowledge and seeking a roadmap to a new you.

You can do this. Remember, enjoy the process. Enjoy your mind and body changing. Enjoy this journey because there are exciting times ahead.

Chapter 8

Nutrition pt1: Calories & Macros

Hair looking like wire. Pale skin dotted with spots. My mouth tasting of metal.

Oh and I was a bit of an emotional wreck too. What was this all about? My new diet and fitness approach was supposed to be improving my health - but I was looking and feeling like crap.

This was the situation I ended up in years ago when I went down the route of drastically cutting the amount of calories I was eating each day in an attempt to regain my body shape.

Sure, I was losing weight and the numbers on the scales were all that matter to me at first. But when you're not sleeping properly, look ill, and feel well below par, then you eventually realise that something's not right. Eventually.

Up until that point, my body was giving me serious warning signs that it was malnourished, but my mind convinced me that if I started eating more then I would put weight on. All I could focus on was getting back to the slim version of me before my daughter was born.

One day I decided that I couldn't continue like this. I was exhausted, I was too tired to do anything, and I felt I didn't even have enough time to spend with my daughter.

By that time I reached that breaking point, I had an obsession with food – or lack of. I'm ashamed to admit this now, but if I managed to stay under 1000 calories per day then I actually felt proud of myself.

Years of in-depth research on health and the workings of the body have been a key part of my studies to become a nurse practitioner.

It then became necessary to properly research the best dietary approach that would not only help me achieve my fat loss fitness goals, but ensure I maintained good health too.

It soon became clear that drastic calorie cutting by reducing my food intake was NOT the answer.

Firstly, I was missing out on important vitamins and minerals that are essential for healthy hair, skin, optimal energy levels, and the overall functioning of the body. I needed more high quality, whole foods to nourish my body and keep it healthy

Secondly, I wasn't providing my body with enough fuel for my day and high intensity workouts. This resulted in me slipping into a worryingly low calorie deficit day after day that was leaving me weak and tired.

Drastic Calorie Cutting Is NOT The Only Way To Lose BodyFat

Calories, simply put, are units of energy. Every cell in our bodies, whether it be muscles or organs, require energy to function at an optimal state and if we don't get enough of that energy source, there are negative consequences, such as; losing muscle mass, inability to focus, low energy levels.

How many calories you need on a daily basis depends on your activity levels and resting metabolic rate. Conventional wisdom tells us that middle aged women, with moderate activity level, should aim for around 1800-2000 calories per day.

We all know that using up more calories than you take in results in weight loss, but eating salads for lunch and dinner, or joining extreme diet plans is not the way.

You've also got to factor in the type of exercise you're doing. A typical weight training session can burn 500 calories alone.

And here's the best part: working out with weights as described in earlier chapters keeps your metabolism levels heightened for 12-24 hours after your workout is finished. (Studies have shown that standard cardio exercise like running or aerobics classes don't have this same effect).

Here's how I see it: weight training allows me to eat more food, enjoy more food, and have a healthier relationship with food.

The more tasty whole foods I ate, the healthier and stronger I felt. The more I combined weight training with these increased calories, the better I felt both mentally and physically.

Turned out I didn't need to cut massive amounts of calories in order to be in good shape, I just had to make sensible food choices most of the time.

Guess what? I didn't gain weight, or become big, or bulky. I became healthier, gradually lost the unwanted bodyfat...but developed muscle tone to match.

Over the years, I've found that this massive calorie cutting is adopted in many approaches to losing weight. There are plenty of weight loss programmes that encourage it.

My advice is to avoid this. It may work for a period, but is definitely not the best long-term approach to get in shape and stay that way.

It should always be about balance, after all. Anything that makes you cut your energy source and robs your body of nutrients over a long period of time will do damage to not only your physical health, but emotional well-being too.

So, don't get too caught up on the amount of calories you're consuming and the total you're burning. Personally, I'm generally around the 1800-1900 calories mark on training days and slightly less on non training days.

I also recommend introducing intermittent fasting to help keep bodyfat levels low, and improve your health. But we'll cover this in a separate chapter.

What About Counting Your 'Macros'?

Carbohydrates, fats and protein are also known as macronutrients (or shortened to 'macros' in the fitness world). These are fundamental for our body to perform at its best.

If you listen to the advice in some fitness magazines, or what some fitness coaches preach, you'd think that there's a perfect ratio of macronutrients you should be eating each meal.

i.e. Your plate should be made up 30% protein, 50% carbs, and 20% fat.

And we all know someone who is on a low carb diet these days, thinking that's the best way to a leaner body.

My advice is the same for macronutrients as it is for calories: don't get too focused on the numbers.

What's more important is that you eat a decent amount of all three macronutrients at each meal - and choose from healthy food sources the majority of the time. (Think 'organic', 'free range', 'unprocessed', 'fresh'....).

A sweet potato is a carbohydrate food source. So is a sticky bun. Which one are you going to choose?

A chicken breast cooked at home with seasoning is a tasty protein source. So chicken covered in breadcrumbs and fried at your local KFC restaurant. Which one will you pick?

Avocados and nuts are a great source of healthy fats. The fat in donuts or French fries is not quite so healthy. I think you get the idea.

And of course, cooking at home using those types of ingredients instead of microwave meals, sweets and treats, and other processed junk, are essential to helping you reach your fitness goals.

How Much Protein?

We all know that protein is essential for muscle development, and is needed for repairing the body after your workouts.

But that simply doesn't mean that more protein = more progress.

If you eat too much protein, your body will not metabolise it effectively. This can have a detrimental effect on your kidneys, and also stress your digestive system.

If you want to figure it out by numbers then try and aim for around 0.7g-1g of protein per pound of body weight.

So, if you weigh 150lbs, you would shoot for roughly 100-150g of protein per day. If you were 160lbs, then around 110-160g per day.

These are ballpark figures and you could still achieve your fitness goals with a lesser amount.

Experiment and see what works best for you.

Pre and Post-Workout Nutrition

There's a big misconception out there that you need bananas, pasta, or even worse, energy drinks, to have plenty of fuel for your gym workouts.

The reasoning behind this is obvious: these are high in carbohydrates, which will be broken down into glucose to give you energy for training hard.

This makes perfect sense, but there are also some downsides to this. Firstly, your body also has to expend energy when digesting stodgy pasta, or trying to metabolise all the processed garbage you find in energy drinks.

Secondly, you're missing out on an ideal fat loss opportunity. By feeding your body with carbs, that will be your body's primary source of energy. However, if you changed things up and lifted weights in the morning with no food beforehand, then your body will use up its fat stores for energy.

The glucose derived from your food intake is converted into glycogen and stored in the body. But when you fast for long periods (i.e. during the night when you're sleeping and not having breakfast too) then that glycogen runs out, and your body will break down fat in the body to use as an energy source.

Pre-workout

While it's not possible for all women to go to the gym in the morning, especially if you have kids or work early, it is a smart move to do so without eating any breakfast.

A black coffee is allowed as the caffeine will definitely give you an energy boost, but leave out the sugar, sweeteners or milk as these will raise your blood sugar levels again and interfere with the fat burning process.

I also use creatine monohydrate, which is a natural supplement that helps increase energy and strength levels. Creatine boosts the production of adenosine triphosphate (ATP), which is basically the body's energy currency. More ATP = working out longer and stronger.

I also take branch chain amino acids tablets as a helpful, but not essential supplement. Amino acids are the building block of protein and are therefore important in the muscle repair and development process.

Post-workout

Post-workout nutrition doesn't have to be complicated. Sure, it will help you move towards your fitness goals if you use a good quality protein powder supplement after each workout.

By drinking a protein shake after you leave the gym you'll be providing your body with an ideal amount of protein, along with simple carbohydrates, and some other nutrients required for the muscle repair and development.

However, you could head home or to the work canteen and eat a nice balanced meal of salmon, potatoes and green veg, and still supply your body with what it needs.

This type of lifestyle is only as complicated as you make it. If you put in hard work and effort then it will become the norm for you, but again, don't put too much pressure on yourself to change everything instantly. Any progress is good progress.

Remember the wall building story? You've got it in you to make these simple changes and I believe you can do it.

Chapter 9

Nutrition pt2: Maintaining a Healthy Diet

Have you come across the fitness hero that is David Goggins yet? If you haven't already read his book Can't Hurt Me, then I'd advise you grab a copy soon.

In his amazing book, Goggins talks about his 40% Rule…which is basically that when you think you've given our all in fitness – whether that's in the gym, running, swimming etc – you've actually only given about 40%. There's so much more you can give and achieve.

Well, I've got a rule too. It's called the 80% Rule…and it means you should be eating healthy, wholesome foods 80% of the time.

You've got to be realistic when it comes to diet and nutrition. My view on clean eating isn't all chicken breast and broccoli for dinner seven days per week.

Rather, eating healthy for me is a reduction in refined sugars and processed meals, and trying to eat natural, whole foods _most_ of the time.

That means preparing healthy dinners and lunches most days of the week, but still enjoying occasional treats and trips to restaurants etc. You've still got to live a little.

You don't have to be a chef to be able to cook tasty, healthy meals and snacks. There are millions of simple and easy recipes available for free online.

I'm going to list my top 10 clean eating tips to help you adopt a healthier approach to nutrition, but first I want to share how things used to go down when I was overweight and unfit.

My previous diet years ago: every Sunday night I convinced myself that I was going to eat healthy the next day. That was my intention and I was sticking to it.

I'd get up and have fruit for breakfast but before long, the sugar cravings started. I'd tell myself that if I just had one unhealthy snack I'd be good for the rest of the day.

For some reason it never quite worked out that way, I lost count of the amount of Sundays where I went round in the same circle.

I knew the food I was eating was unhealthy, but I was so uneducated on what was right for me. Everywhere I looked it was either 'low calorie', 'low fat', 'no fat', 'low sugar', 'low carb'. It was a minefield.

During this time I was also very low mentally, like most of us are at some point in our lives, I was going through a pretty difficult time and was comfort eating. The sweet stuff made me feel better, for a time, but then I ended up feeling worse.

I was gaining more and more weight which in turn, was making me feel even worse. It was a negative loop.

Eat More Of This, Eat Less Of That...

For the past five years or so my nutrition has changed dramatically, and it's been much easier than I thought. My dietary intake consists of mainly whole foods, a lot of fresh fruit and vegetables, nuts, and some lean cuts of meat.

My ex-partner Marc and I made a conscious decision to reduce the amount of meat in our diet due to several reasons including factory farming, food quality, and improving our health.

While I do still eat meat three or four days per week, this switch meant that we were cooking a lot more fresh, plant-based meals and snacks.

And last year, we published a recipe book filled our favourite recipes called 'The Meat Free Fitness Menu: 51 Healthy Vegetarian Recipes For Gym Lovers'.

While my meat intake has vastly reduced over the past year, that's simply a personal choice. I'm certainly not trying to convince you to do the same.

Below is an overall basic guide as to which foods and drinks to eat more of, and which ones to avoid or at least limit throughout the week.

Foods To Eat

All kinds of vegetables (ideally organic), fruit, nuts, nut butters, chicken, lean meats, pulses, free range eggs, fish, oats and oatcakes, Greek yoghurt, rice, plant-based protein powder, dark chocolate and various spices to flavour your food (i.e. oregano, turmeric, cinnamon, ginger).

Foods To Avoid/Limit

Microwave ready meals, high sugar foods (cakes, chocolate, ice cream, desserts etc), high sugar drinks (all fizzy sodas like cola, lemonade, energy drinks etc), fast food/takeaway meals, and basically highly-processed foods.

Cooking fresh is always the best step, then you know you're not consuming processed garbage. There are thousands of great recipe books out there, and a ton of free recipes available on websites and blogs just by doing a basic Google search.

Generally speaking, if you're going to buy anything pre-packed then a good rule of thumb to adopt is; anything with more than six ingredients on the packaging is best avoided – most of the time.

Don't take the easy step and buy in processed junk from the supermarket, get cooking with some of the countless tasty recipes you can make yourself.

Nowadays, the food choices I make leave me feeling nourished, full, and give me plenty of energy most days. This creates a positive feedback loop where I don't feel bagged up and heavy, and I'm proud of myself for resisting the junk and nourishing my body.

Don't get me wrong, it's not easy to simply switch to a healthy diet if you've struggled with a sweet tooth, or alcohol, or easy takeaway meals for years. It's not done easily – but it CAN be done.

7 Tips For Maintaining A Healthy Diet

#1 Remember the 80% Rule

This means eating clean most of the time, not all of the time. It's okay to have a cheat day. And it's okay to have a little chocolate now and again, don't be guilt tripping yourself over this kind of stuff.

#2 Get cooking

I cook fresh meals for dinner and make enough for lunch the next day too. I do this all throughout the week, which guarantees that at least two of my 3 meals per day are super healthy.

#3 Find healthy snack alternatives

Snacking on sweet treats and crisps etc after dinner or watching the TV is where most of us struggle, right? Especially after a long day at work.

But if you snack on junk like this every weeknight, it's all going to add up. Instead, find healthy snack alternatives. Mine is dark chocolate (70% or above), which is healthy and low in sugar, or look up some healthy snack recipes online and have them instead.

#4 Follow intermittent fasting

As long as you're doing intermittent fasting properly, it means your body is burning fat automatically. While this doesn't give you the green light for more unhealthy food choices, it does give you peace of mind that the occasional treat isn't going to go straight to your hips.

#5 Think about how hard you've worked in the gym

Usually when you start craving junk food it's all about instant gratification, and satisfying a need there and then. To help overcome that craving, think about how hard you've been working in the gym...many hours over weeks and months.

Then consider the fact that you could enhance those efforts with a healthier option, or sabotage them with a quick sugar fix.

#6 Think about how you'll feel afterwards

I don't know about you, but 90% of the time after I stuff my face with a greasy takeaway meal I feel like crap afterwards. Bloated, sluggish, and needing a nap. That feeling says it all about your body struggling to break down so much rubbish. Maybe if you consider that horrible feeling before ordering the 14 inch pizza, you'll think again.

#7 Spice things up

This point actually ties in #2 and cooking fresh. Just because you're eating more whole foods and plenty of vegetables and fruit, doesn't mean your meals have to be boring and tasteless.

By stocking up on plenty of spices, such as oregano, turmeric, paprika, chilli powder etc, you can give your meals a real kick – and plenty of flavour.

These are just some basic pieces of advice but will certainly help you implement a healthier nutritional lifestyle.

Eating good = feeling good = feeling more confident + continuing to nourish your body.

Remember, it's a gradual process. Don't be too harsh on yourself if you have some slip-ups at first, at least you're trying. It's taken me six years of continual changes and tweaking things, not to mention tons of research to adopt this approach.

There's so much information out there that it can leave you feeling overwhelmed. Eating a good balanced diet strengthens the mind, it boost your self-worth, and then it does get easier to make more appropriate food choices in future.

Remember The Important Stuff…

- Eat clean 80% of the time
- Cut down on refined sugar and processed, pre-packed meals.
- Avoid extreme calorie cutting.
- If you choose pre-packed items – aim for something with six ingredients or less.
- Enjoy nourishing your body and mind. Your body will thank you for it in the long run.
- If you want a sweet treat or a takeaway occasionally then have it, just know that you have the mental strength to go back to the good stuff.

Eat a nice healthy, balanced diet 80% of the time. That doesn't mean going absolutely nuts at the weekend and gorging down as much junk food as possible.

But if you want a takeaway and a beer then have it. If you have a long overdue night out with the girls, then have it, guilt free.

Just always make sure you're back on track the next day. But please, please, please, I cannot stress this enough, don't put too much pressure on yourself to change everything at once.

You'll undoubtedly hate the journey - and life in general! Just approach it sensibly like any new task…small changes every day. Your hard work and effort will pay off.

Also, don't be put off thinking that you won't have enough time to cook healthy meals. Working full time and bringing up my daughter on my own, I initially got stressed even thinking about where I'd find the time to prepare all the healthy food.

It's simply all about being organised, and us women are great multi-taskers. By cooking bigger portions at dinner time, you can also fix tomorrow's lunch with the leftovers. And some healthy meals can be whipped up in 15-20 mins.

Don't listen to all the people pushing extreme diet plans or telling you to count every calorie. Adopting – and maintaining – a healthy diet is easier than you think.

Bonus Healthy Snack Recipes

Like I mentioned earlier, I know that unhealthy snacking is a common pitfall for most of us. Chocolate or biscuits after dinner, or desserts and other sweet treats, are bad habits that can be hard to break.

I've already advised that you find healthy alternatives, such as dark chocolate. But, as a wee bonus from your pal Vicki, I've included a couple of healthy snack recipes below that are included in my 'Meat Free Fitness Menu' recipe book. Enjoy!

No Bake Protein Balls

These little balls of brilliance are so easy to make as there's no cooker involved.

Simply gather the ingredients, mix them up, and get rollin' into healthy snacks you eat at home - or take with you in a tub to work.

Ingredients	**Servings – 8**
2 scoops chocolate protein powder	
100g rolled oats	**Nutrition Per**
1 tsp cinnamon	**Serving**
4 tbsp cup smooth nut butter	
3 tsp natural honey	**Calories: 158**
1 tsp vanilla extract	**Protein: 9g**
30g raisins	**Carbs: 20g**
50ml almond milk	**Fat: 5g**

Serving Instructions

Step 1

Add oats, protein powder, and cinnamon to a large bowl.

Step 2

Add in peanut butter, honey and vanilla extract. Stir to combine.

Step 3

Pour in raisins next and stir through. Mixture should be slightly sticky but still crumbly.

Step 4

Slowly add in liquid 1 tablespoon at a time and, using your hands, combine until it comes together in a sticky ball that holds together.

If mixture is too dry, add in more liquid but not so much that it won't hold shape.

Step 5

Roll into balls using hands, and then place in a container to set in the fridge for at least 30 mins. After that time, they're good to go!

Chocolate & Peanut Oats

This simple recipe is ready in just 5 mins.

Ingredients
40g oats
300ml almond milk
½ scoop chocolate protein powder
(MyProtein Vegan Blend)
1 tbsp organic natural peanut butter
½ banana (optional)

Servings – 1

Nutrition Per Serving
Calories: 509
Protein: 32g
Carbs: 60g
Fat: 24g

Cooking Instructions

Step 1

Add oats and milk into a bowl and stir to combine.

Step 2

Microwave for 1 minute, then stir and continue to microwave in 30 second increments, stirring between each, until the oatmeal is the consistency you like.

Step 3

Mash the banana and add to the oats.

Step 4

Carefully remove from microwave. Mix the protein powder into the oats, stirring thoroughly until completely dissolved. Finally, top with peanut butter.

Chapter 10

Nutrition pt3: Intermittent Fasting

Have you heard of intermittent fasting before now? If not, do you think it means starving yourself?

That was my first reaction. The word fasting scared me. I thought fasting = starving.

I thought, like many people do, that this must be a crazy new diet trend where you hardly eat anything to get skinny.

I wanted to eat effectively to support my weight training but I had moved away from the fad diet gang, I didn't want to go back to restricting what and how much I ate.

I had been spending months researching the best eating approach to help with my weight loss and intermittent fasting kept popping up.

I discovered it meant having a long break without food in your day in order to experience numerous health and fat loss benefits.

As a busy, single mum, working full time, I was finding it difficult to eat smaller meals every few hours like is often recommended by fitness trainers. So intermittent fasting definitely appealed to me. I needed something that supported my lifestyle, as well as my weight loss and weightlifting programme.

Turns out my judgmental mind had it all wrong at first. Intermittent fasting - or IF as it's often referred - allows for a much more relaxed approach to eating healthy.

And far from starving yourself, I only apply one simple rule...don't eat breakfast.

With all the research I'd done, I felt I had enough knowledge to implement this new diet approach, so I started it slowly.

there's tonnes of research out there on how to do this, the 16:8 method, the 5:2 way, or alternate day fasting.

I found what worked best for me was to fast for no longer than 14 hours, and have a 10 hour eating window. If the thought of this is scaring you a little, that's okay, no need to worry.

Let me explain: out of those 14 hours, you're going to be sleeping for around 7-9 of them. Unless you're some crazy human who has the ability to eat while sleeping, then this may be difficult for you.

You get up in the morning and, if time allows it, you get to the gym for a workout and eat afterwards. It's really that simple.

Not only that but studies show that this method of eating is actually sooooo good for your overall health and wellbeing.

You see, if you eat before training, you use those calories to fuel your workout - which means any energy used will come from that recent meal to use for fuel.

If you fast for longer than 10 hours, the body automatically goes to your glycogen stores for energy. But when these run out, the body is very clever, it'll use your stored fat for future energy needs. So why not use those stores to fuel your workout?

I've spoken to loads of people and the main thing they always say is "I can't train fasted, I wouldn't have the energy", that little voice in your head again, you know the one, the one that likes everything to be comfortable and stay the same.

Remember, nothing changes if nothing changes. Not only does fasting use fat stores to fuel your workout, it also has an amazing ability to increase growth hormone. Arghhhhh sciency stuff!

Growth hormone is produced in a tiny gland in the brain, it's what is used in the body for growth and repair.

It helps children grow taller, but as you get older and taller, the body releases less of this anabolic hormone. But growth hormone also has another amazing job, it's what controls muscle growth and decreases body fat.

Incorporating these two simple changes can regulate your metabolism. Guess what else increases growth hormone? Weight training!

When we lift heavier loads at a greater frequency (less rest time) we cause our bodies to release greater amounts of growth hormone.

Weight training + intermittent fasting = fat burning machine.

Here's a simple way of approaching it, incorporate slowly at first, let your body adjust. Start with this relaxed way of eating two days a week. Eat your dinner at say 8pm, get a workout in the morning, and eat at around 10am the next day.

When you feel comfortable then increase the days, before you know it, this will be your way of eating and you wont even have to look at the time. Again, your body will get so used to it, it's equipped for change and can adjust.

Just silence that voice in your head. You know, that annoying one.

But why 14 hours? Evidence suggests that although fasting has various many health benefits, fasting for more than five days a week at a time for longer than 14 hours can have a detrimental effect on women's menstrual cycles.

I do occasionally fast for longer but that is only now and then. Just make sure you're eating enough calories. Intermittent fasting and calorie restriction is dangerous, a reduction in calories can cause hormonal imbalances, irregular period and increases your risk of infertility.

Tips:

- Do not fast for longer than 24 hours at a time
- Ideally fast for 12 to 16 hours
- Do not restrict calories
- Do not fast on consecutive days during your first two to three weeks of fasting (for instance, if you do a 14 hour fast, do it two days a week instead of seven)
- Drink plenty of fluids during your fast

This dietary method is an amazing way to aid your physical and mental journey. And it's advised not to do it every day. I do intermittent fasting for 5 days out of 7, and that's it.

I do a 14 hour fast Monday to Friday, and then eat normally the other two weekend days, but it's entirely up to you how you work it out.

I find that intermittent fasting allows my diet to be much more relaxed, and less restricted. I still get to see and feel the great benefits it has to offer. But, I get to enjoy having breakfast with my daughter at the weekend.

I'm not going to try to convince you to follow the intermittent fasting approach just because I do, but it is certainly worth researching further. Here are just some of the benefits you'll read about online that make it appealing:

- Can help lose weight and belly fat

- Lowers the risk of type 2 diabetes
- Can reduce overall inflammation in the body
- Beneficial for heart health
- May help prevent cancer
- Can be good for your brain – by increasing the growth of new nerve cells
- May prevent Alzheimer's disease
- Can help you live longer
- Can change the function of cells, genes and hormones
- Boosts energy levels

If those aren't good enough reasons to give it a shot, I don't know what is.

Chapter 11

Love Your Body

We see it everywhere. We long for it...but we can never quite get it.

You know what I'm talking about: the airbrushed women all around us, in magazines, on TV, on billboards. The person you think you want to look like.

Society puts so much pressure on women in terms of appearance. Of course, it's important to look after your physical appearance and your health and wellbeing, but not in such a narrow-minded way.

The only person you should try to measure up against is yourself. I know this sounds very basic, but the more focus you put on yourself, and less on other people around you, the more you will begin to accept yourself and your body.

I don't think that anyone is 100% 'happy' with their body shape. We humans are pretty damn good at always finding fault in something, particularly when it comes to our body shape and appearance.

We're our own worst critics at times, and that's exactly what we've got to change.

Sure, we all want less bodyfat and more muscle tone. And the weight training and nutrition approaches shared in this book WILL absolutely help you achieve this.

But I want to make it clear that the main focus of this book is about helping you become stronger physically and mentally, and improving your health and wellbeing.

Too often, the aesthetics side of things and being "unhappy" with our bum, "hating" the cellulite on our legs, or "wishing to change" the flab on our arms is what's really holding us back.

The fitness journey is about acceptance. It's about testing yourself and developing your self-esteem. And it's ultimately about becoming more accepting and compassionate towards yourself.

It's time to stop worrying about what other people think. It's time to stop comparing ourselves to others.

It's time to start loving our bodies more.

When I first started out lifting weights, I had one goal, and one goal only...to lose weight. I wasn't happy with my body, I felt so disappointed in myself every time I looked in the mirror or saw pictures of myself.

I actually avoided having photos taken due to how uncomfortable I felt when I looked at them afterwards. I wasn't in a good place mentally or physically. I thought back then that if I became fit and lost weight, then I'd be happy.

I thought being thin was the route to happiness. Very superficial, I know.

My weight training regime and new nutritional approach did make me happy but not in the way I thought it would.

The more I lifted weights, the stronger I became, and it motivated me to start setting personal goals. For every goal I achieved I became more confident and focused, which made me enjoy life more, which in turn made me view myself and my body in an entirely different way.

Positive feedback loop.

I honestly believe that if I hadn't faced my fears in the beginning about lifting weights in the once-daunting gym environment, then I wouldn't have become the person I am today.

The dedication, commitment and discipline that comes with a proper workout programme changes your mindset. It also helped me put things in perspective and appreciate what I've got more, rather than dwelling on insecurities.

I have an amazing job, amazing daughter and amazing life. That's what's important.

Lifting weights not only changes your physical appearance, it makes you mentally strong, and far more likely you'll achieve goals outside of the gym too, but I believe it sets a healthy example for those closest to you, particularly your children.

There's a little quote that I feel resonates here: "There is no limit to what we, as women, can accomplish". I wholeheartedly believe that we can do anything we set our minds to. Me six years ago would never have believed that.

Lift Weights...And Lift Your Entire Life

I'll be honest, I once hated my life. I often woke up in the morning with a horrible feeling in my stomach, and I tried to make it shift by distracting myself with other things.

I felt bad as I had a beautiful daughter, a roof over my head, and a job. Why couldn't I just be happy? I'd beat myself up over simple things. I'd put pressure on myself to be what others expected of me.

Lifting weights has changed all of that. It's made me a more assertive person. It's given me the confidence to make important decisions which influence the lives of myself and my daughter.

You see, it's not all physical with weight training. The benefits go far beyond that. You also build mental toughness, you somehow develop better coping mechanisms, and resilience for what life throws at you.

By pushing yourself hard in the gym, and overcoming the many excuses not to do so, you gradually acquire all these new qualities.

That's exactly what happened to me. That's exactly what's happened to numerous friends I meet in the gym. So I know it can be the same for you too.

I always thought achievers were people who were lucky in life. But if you put in the physical effort required at the gym consistently, and consistently stretch your limits, then you can achieve anything you put your mind to

Being part of the fad diet crowd is not sustainable. You always feel restricted and, while your willpower can hold out for a while, it never lasts; not to mention the damage it can do to your health and metabolism in the long term.

For me, fad diets and cutting calories had my emotions all over the place, which made me go back to the unhealthy foods to try and feel better temporarily...which of course made me miserable as soon as I stopped eating.

It was a no-win situation that cycled for years, and again I was back to hating my body shape. Fortunately, I don't even recognise that person now and I'm so grateful for that.

Lifting weights has completely changed my view of my body and mind. If I gain a few pounds here and there, so what? I have the confidence now to accept and love my body the way it is.

I go on holiday and enjoy all the tasty food options. I go out for dinner and eat what I want. I go to the cinema and order large popcorn, and I have nights out and never count calories.

Weight training, intermittent fasting, making sensible food choices, and avoiding fad diets is what makes all this possible.

I love my life, and I truly believe that I would never have been this way if I didn't start weight training. My mind is strong and focused, I know I will never go back to the mindset I had six years ago.

If I can do this then so can you. You know you can, and it all starts with facing that first fear. Your future self will thank you for it.

If you're not happy with where you're at physically and mentally today, then sure be realistic about your current position and the serious effort you're going to have to put in to improve yourself.

But take on the challenge from a strong position of loving your body and loving yourself. No self-criticisms, or labels, or negative chatter in your head. Don't allow any space for that.

Instead, be focused, determined, hard-working, self-accepting, and a good role model for your children or people you love around you.

That's how you become Stronger Than Ever.

Conclusion

I'm super proud of you. Not only for taking this step and buying the book, but for being dedicated to change.

You've given your valuable time reading about all my struggles, pitfalls, and insecurities that I promise you I've never shared until now.

I did go on a bit, but I felt I had to be completely honest about everything I had gone through to get to this positive place, a place I know you can get to.

You've committed yourself to starting something very important and I'm excited for what could lay ahead for you. My only hope is that you stay committed to seeing this through...as this is just the start of your journey.

What now? Apply that commitment and work hard in the gym, but importantly be patient. Your results won't come in a few weeks, but they will come if you keep taking action, and believe in yourself.

And remember, you don't have to completely overhaul your diet or struggle to eat healthy all the time. Just 80% of the time will do nicely, and you can't still have treats from time to time.

All the guidance in the previous chapters on diet and training are just words of course. They mean completely nothing unless followed up with action. The onus is now on you to move things forward.

The 13 fundamental exercises and the 13 extras will give you amazing results in the gym. You'll become much stronger physically and can transform your body shape, but I hope the benefits go far beyond that for you.

I hope it boosts your self-esteem like it did for me, and I hope it supercharges you to gain extra confidence outside of the gym too.

Just always remember, don't put too much pressure on yourself. And don't try to change every detail at once, as you'll end up hating this fitness journey...and life in general.

Make the necessary changes based on what you've learned. Build that wall brick by brick, but try to enjoy that process of change. Weight training and becoming a stronger you should be fun.

Most fitness books I've read only really discuss diet and exercise, but I wanted this book to be a bit different. I wanted it to be real and to be able to connect with other women who have a whole host of things going on.

Working full time, having children, trying to remember every bloody detail of everything.

Adding a complex training and diet plan to that mix will only result in failure. That's why the methods in this book are easy to implement into your life, and they're easy to maintain over the long haul.

Every part of this book is just as important as the other; exercise routines, dietary advice, applying yourself, facing your fears, developing a strong mindset and learning to love your body.

All of these components go hand in hand, and if you apply all of them I KNOW you'll see results, mentally, physically and emotionally.

You have got it in you to take your lifestyle to the next level. If you're dedicated and committed to change then your halfway there.

I'm backing you all the way, and I'm happy to offer any advice on anything you're unsure about. Feel free to send me an email any time at: **vicki@vic-fit.com**

Now put down the book - and get ready for some serious action.

Acknowledgments

This book would not have been possible without a few special people.

Firstly, my dad who passed away when I was 20 years old. I was devastated but without his guidance and wisdom, I would never have become the person I am today. His death also made me realise that life's too short.

My beautiful daughter Ciara. She is my entire world and the one who has kept me going through tough times in the past. She probably doesn't realise the impact she has on my life, and I'm so proud of the person she's becoming.

My mum, the most caring and supportive woman I know.

My good friend Marc. He has not only helped me get this book out there, but has also pushed me when doubt has set in. He's also great at coming up with excellent ideas during hiking expeditions.

Finally, J. He keeps me focused and balanced. Not only that, but he reminds me to trust the journey that is life. Thank you.

ABOUT THE AUTHOR

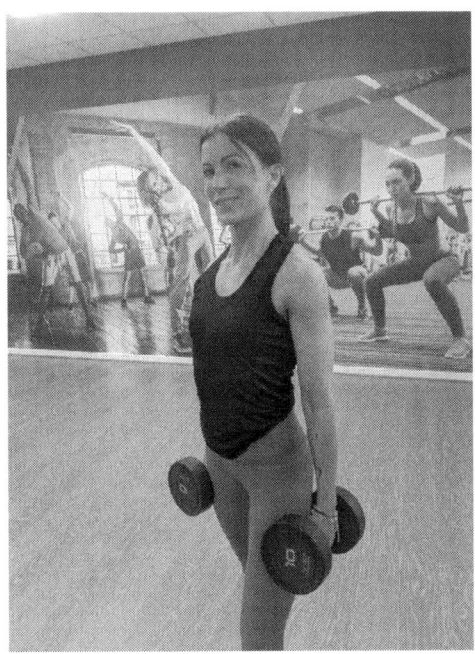

Victoria Murphy is a 37-year-old mum to Ciara, and lives in West Dunbartonshire, Scotland.

Currently working as an Advanced Nurse Practitioner at a hospital near Glasgow, Victoria is interested in all things health, fitness and wellness.

Her hobbies enjoy eating, hillwalking, camping, yoga, eating, acting stupid, singing badly, and eating.

Victoria's website is: **www.vic-fit.com**

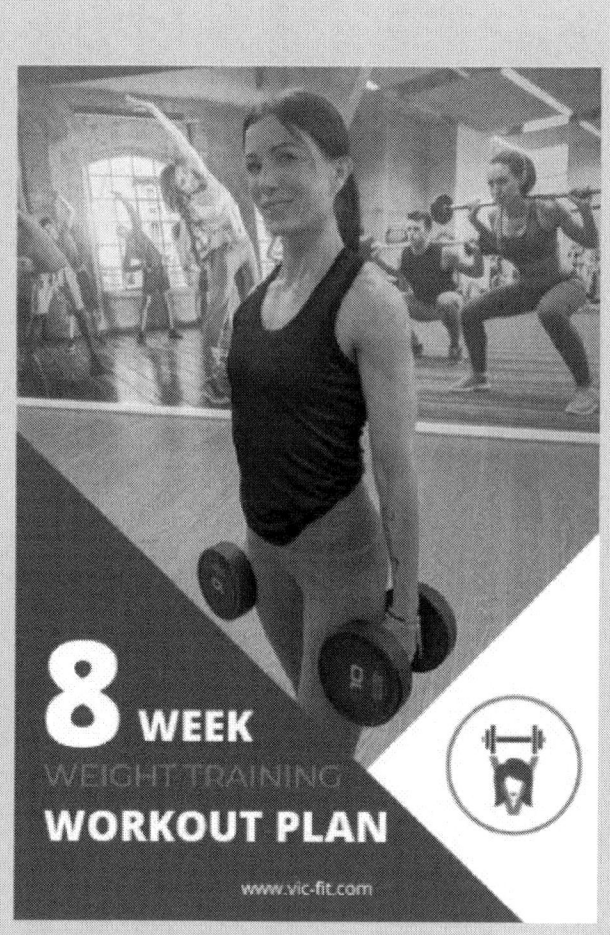

Would you like my 8-week
gym workout plan for free?
Grab your copy at:
www.vic-fit.com

Printed in Great Britain
by Amazon

53617611R00093